Aging and the Nervous System

Aging and the
Nervous System

Salvatore Giaquinto
Hospital of San Giovanni Battista, Rome, Italy

A Wiley Medical Publication

JOHN WILEY & SONS
Chichester · New York · Brisbane · Toronto · Singapore

Library of Congress Cataloging-in-Publication Data
Giaquinto, Salvatore.
    Aging and the nervous system/Salvatore Giaquinto.
       p.   cm. — (A Wiley medical publication)
    ISBN 0 471 91835 0
    1. Nervous system — Aging.   2. Geriatrics.   I. Title.   II. Series.
    [DNLM: 1. Aging.   2. Brain Diseases — in old age.   3. Nervous
    System — physiopathology.   WL 102 G434a]
QP361.B54 1988
612'.8 — dc19
DNLM/DLC
for Library of Congress   87-37183
                                                                     CIP

British Library Cataloguing in Publication Data
Giaquinto, Salvatore
    Aging and the nervous system.
    1. Geriatric neurology   2. Nervous system
    — Aging
    I. Title
    612'.8   RC346

    ISBN 0 471 91835 0

Phototypeset in Times by Ellis Horwood Limited
Printed and bound in Great Britain by Anchor Brendon Ltd., Colchester, Essex

Contents

to my parents

Foreword

The Order of the Knights of Malta sponsors medical research and health care in many countries, continuing a charitable tradition whose history goes back a thousand years. Today, in our hospitals around the world, we are discovering the importance of rehabilitation programmes, particularly in the treatment of elderly patients. Advances in health care have prolonged the average life span: now we must ensure that the quality of that life is maintained.

Professor Salvatore Giaquinto is chief neurologist at the Hospital of San Giovanni Battista (St John the Baptist) in Rome, one of the many hospitals run by the Order in Italy. Here he has led the medical team responsible for the development of intensive and remarkably effective new programmes of rehabilitation for elderly patients suffering from disorders of the nervous system. In this initiative, medical research has gone hand-in-hand with patient care.

Professor Giaquinto's monograph describes the structural and neuropsychological changes which take place in the aging nervous system, in health and in disease. He considers the techniques which may be used to maintain the quality of life in the normal aged, and to rehabilitate those in whom the brain is damaged. Professor Giaquinto is particularly concerned with the relationship between aging and dementia, and the problems raised by the increasing incidence of this condition in the population. He has written this book with the intention of making the medical and social issues accessible to the general reader as well as to the clinician.

On behalf of the Knights of Malta, I welcome this publication which reflects the human values and medical care which the Order strives to promote throughout the world.

Carlo Marullo di Condojanni
Commissario Magistrale dell'Associazione dei Cavalieri Italiani del
    Sovrano Militare Ordine di Malta
Palazzo de Grillo, Rome

Acknowledgements

Thanks are due to Drs Cornelio Fazio, Franco Angeleri, Stuart Butler, Veeramani Maharajan, Menotti Calvani and Giuseppe Nolfe for their helpful discussion, respectively, on clinical neurology, neuropsychology, neuroanatomy, genetics, pharmacology and statistics. The author is also grateful to Dr Stuart Butler for the revision of the text. Thanks are also due to Dr Adelaide Pietraroja and Miss Cristina De Montis for the preparation of the manuscript and to Mr Franco Orlandi for his drawings.

The publication of this book was made possible through the generous support of Sigma-Tau Pharmaceuticals, Rome.

CHAPTER 1

Myth, culture and religion

There is disagreement over whether Man has always resisted the idea of Old Age.

Old age has always fascinated and terrified mankind. It has been said that when it is on the horizon, everyone looks forward to old age, but when it arrives aging becomes a thing to be resisted.

One of the most important contributions that a study of literature can give us is the ability to see how man has tried to understand the idea of his own decay. Thousands of years of literary observation compensate for the lack of scientific . and statistical data. Literature has, therefore, scientific value.

In the classical era we find that the concept of death was more acceptable than the idea of old age. This is illustrated in the myth of Aurora. Aurora fell in love with Thiton, a young Trojan. She implored Zeus to grant her lover eternal life. Her wish was fulfilled but, as she did not ask for eternal *youth*, Thiton is condemned to an eternal state of senility until he begs Zeus to rid him of his sad condition.

The Greek playwright Menander, on the other hand abandoned mythology in order to concentrate on scenes of real life in his work for the theatre. He follows Euripides in his study of human passion and psychological interaction. Some fragments of his incompleted work curse old age.

Old Age is symbolic of trouble and sorrow

1

and:

Old Age bears with it anger and misery

One of his most famous maxims — apparently paradoxical — runs:

Those whom the Gods love, die young

This means that those who die young escape the burdens of senile decay (and the corruption of old age).

Even in Greek lyric poetry a feeling of catastrophe is conveyed; a few of Mimnermus' lines make it clear how disastrous it is that Zeus has created old age. Another Greek poet, Anacreontes, sighs of love for a young woman but:

She who comes from the fair houses of Lesbos is repelled by my white hair and sighs eagerly for another (man).

Alcmene, himself a lyric poet, tells the lovely young women singers that his body is no longer able to sustain him and that he would love to turn into a bird, free to touch the waves of the sea. Of all Greek tragic playrights Euripides is the most modern. In his tragedy *Alcestis,* Admetus rages at his father who, like his mother, does not wish to die in his place. He adds that none should believe the old, who always beg for death to come to them, but when it does, they cling to this life.

Aristotle, who, as a physician's son, was always intrigued by nature, observes that in order to enjoy a happy old age, people should be free from illness and infirmities. As an accurate observer, he notices that old people are often bad-tempered, selfish and suspicious.

Aristophanes, a writer of Greek comedy, and Plautus in Rome both introduce the stock character of the doddering elder who has lost his memory. This character invariably becomes the butt of laughter and derision. The most famous latin tag on this theme is from Terence:

Senectus ipsa morbus est

says Cremetes, who has been delayed by illness. He is explaining to his astonished brother that old age is itself a disease. Cicero's famous line is a lament that old age is a much heavier burden to bear than the volcano Etna itself:

Ut onus Aetna gravius dicant sustinere senectutem

In the Latin world even Seneca curses; as:

Old age is an incurable disease

and the poet Juvenal abandons his satirical tone to comment bitterly on the absence of comfort and the numerous troubles which attend old age:

Senectus nullo cum commodo venit sed quam continuis et quantis longa senectute plena malis

Shakespeare, speaking through the character of Jaques who has retired to nature in the Ardennes, comments on the last sad scene of the seven ages of man:

Last scene of all
that ends this strange eventual history,
is second childishness, and mere oblivion,
sans teeth, sans eyes, sans taste, sans everything.

The poet Robert Burns, who died when he was 37, expresses his worries about the changes that occur after the age of 45 (quoted by Katzman, 1983)

For ance that five-and-forty's speel'd
see crasy, weary joyless Eild,
Wi wrinkled face
comes hostin' hirplin' owre the field
Wi creepin' pace.

In the rather more colourful atmosphere of nineteenth-century Rome, the poet Belli describes the ravages of age in a masterful sonnet. Translation has softened the raw original but there is still some realistic description

Come and see my grandmother's beauty. She has got ten inches of skin under the goitre, she is rugged like a loaf and shakes like a leaf. She has no more teeth to eat a piece of bread. Her eyes disappear into a round hole, while her nose converges towards her chin. Her arms and legs seem to be fan sticks. Her voice sounds like a frog. Her breasts are a couple of small sacks, but my grandmother was beautiful in her youth. Give time to time and, my dear wife, you will become worse than her.

The poet does not stop at the physical transformation of old age, but he also lists the psychological changes in another sonnet.

Suspicious, lunatic, stubborn with strange ideas and more prickly than thistles

The elegant and solitary Goethe talks through the voice of Faust (Act 1) who has resigned himself to the sadness of old age:

However I dress, I shall feel the pain of such a miserly existence

An Italian poet, Gabriele d'Annunzio (1863–1938) who was not only a refined aesthete but a staunch worshipper of art, defines old age as 'human ruin that is worse than putrefaction'. In the novel *The Fire,* he tells the story of the Countess Radiana, who in Venice

when on a too-light morning realized that the winter of age had begun, decided to leave the world rather than show the ruin of her beauty.

It is also possible to identify in literature from classical times up to the present day at least nine different forms of a distinct gerontological humour (Kehl, 1985). They are: the foibles of frustrating ages *sui generis* (for example, 'the average American woman is not old at forty; in fact, she isn't even forty'); expressions of what it means to grow old (for example, 'an old man gives good advice in order to console himself for no longer being in condition set to set a bad example'); the relativity of age (for example, 'he was either a man of about 150 who was rather young for his years or a man of about 110 who had been aged by trouble'); physical decline (for example, 'as a man gets older, he suspects that nature organized him for the benefit of dentists and doctors'); mental decline (for example, 'you know that you are old when you forget names and then just forget; when you forget to pull up your zipper and then forget to pull it down'); social relationship (for example, 'being an old maid is like death by drowning: a really delightful sensation after you cease to struggle'); youth and age (for example, 'in youth we run into difficulties, whereas in old age difficulties run into us'); black humour (for example, 'the geriatric hotel is a local airport, where are gathered those about to depart into the heavens'); shattering of old age stereotypes (for example, 'the story is told of Mr Holmes at eighty-five, out walking with a friend. When they saw a beautiful young lady, Mr Holmes was heard to sigh "Oh, to be seventy again"').

Most of the authors quoted above seem to have condemned the condition of old age forever. At different places and times, they have described the putrid ruin of humanity in both prose and verse! The reader may infer that the portrayal of age in classical literature — and painting too (the caricatures of Holbein, for example) — is essentially negative.

However, we can point to a parallel tradition in literature and painting which sings the praises of age and the elderly: 'The Mothers's Portrait' by Giacomo Balla (1874–1958) (see the back cover) is full of solemnity rather than regret.

In the classical era, Solon, one of the Seven Sages who lived to be ninety, says that a man should never cease learning, even in old age. Sophocles, whose son attempted to have him put away, recited his tragedy *Oedipus at Colonus* from memory to prove that he was in full possession of his mental powers. Plato in *The Republic* has elders to rule the city and Cato regards the pursuit of virtue as the highest mental activity. The famous sophist Gorgie lived to the age of 102 with his mental agility intact.

If we examine the *Divine Comedy* from this point of view — Dante's masterpiece, blending culture, faith and the beliefs of the thirteenth century — we find many old people who are anything but senile. The first to be mentioned is Charon, the boatman of Hades who transfers damned souls across the river Styx. He is vigorous, with white hair and flaming eyes. He shows his vigour by hitting any slacking oarsman. If the thirteenth century image of old age had been associated with senility, Dante would have surely used another literary model.

Again, in the *Inferno* Dante portrays the old tailor who doggedly tries to thread his needle to follow his trade despite many difficulties. There are more venerable old gentlemen of great stature to be found in the *Divine Comedy*. Cato stands guard at the foot of the mountain in purgatory as a symbol of moral authority. On top of the mountain, two dignified old men represent the *Acts of the Apostles* and the *Letters of St Paul,* while a third solitary old man lies asleep, symbolizing the *Revelation of St John.* A final reference which is, perhaps the most relevant, is that Dante is accompanied on his journey first by Virgil (poetry) and then Beatrice (faith) but neither are judged as competent to plead before God. They are replaced by St Bernard of Clairvaux. The allegory is very clear: for the best approach to God, the person's gift should be refined through the maturity of old age.

Another Catholic writer who describes the vigour of the old is Alessandro Manzoni (1785–1873). Here is his respectful portrayal of Cardinal Borromeo:

The habit of solemn and benevolent thinking, the internal peace of a long life, love of mankind and continuous joy in future hope had substituted, I should say, an aged beauty.

To end this personal collection of literary references concerning old age, I shall mention the admiration of the Italian philosopher Vincenzo Gioberti (1801–1852), for:

the Christian old age is full of honour and calm. White hair denotes prophetic authority when it is coupled with a keen mind and the purity of unselfish fame.

I have only reported extracts from the literature I know. Another author (Wertheimer, 1983) who believes in the importance of classical literature in order to understand the concept of old age, cites examples from French literature. Every reader has probably collected a series of literary quotations, folk tales, popular songs and sayings from his own country. It may prove impossible to achieve a complete collection. Even if the work is incomplete at present a conclusion does emerge from an examination of these pieces. In cultures, like the classical, which are based on physical and productive capabilities as well as heroic and erotic values, old age is seen as a slow and sad decline. In cultures where there is spiritual vision, like the Christian faith, old age is a process of spiritual elevation in the period of earthly life which immediately precedes eternal life. According to this latter view, old age is a solemn and honourable state as Cato's in Dante.

An anthropological study carried out in Kenya (Bahemuka, 1982) shows the esteem in which the old are held. To be called 'old' is a compliment. The elderly hold rank and status in both religious and social activities, particularly in initiation rites.

Old people in African communities accept their age with grace. They are closer to the spirits than the young and will seek revenge after death if they are not respected on earth. The spirits of the tribe's ancestors exercise a controlling influence on the living. Belief in reincarnation reduces the difference between life and death.

Social customs transmit a code of obedience to the old. The respect for the elderly in this type of society reminds us of an episode in Ancient Greece. During the Olympic Games, an old Athenian was looking for a seat among his fellow-citizens, without success. When he passed the seats taken by the rival Spartans, they, to a man, stood up to offer him a seat.

Among the Australian Aborigines the word 'old' is synonymous with 'great' ('Ke-Turkekai' in the language of the Kowregara). The 'great man' has the pick of the youngest and prettiest girls, leaving the uglier girls to the younger men.

Other peoples, from New Caledonia, or the North American Indians have the same high regard for the old. In Samoa, the elderly receive deference and respectful treatment from the younger members of society. The experience of the older adults entitles them to be advisors on the resources and activities of the village. Although recent developments were expected to reduce the status of old people, the family setting and culture have protected the traditional values and regard for the old (Rhoads, 1984).

In Papua a person becomes 'old' when his parents die or when he can no longer look after himself, or when the first nephew is born. Old people have great influence. Their reduced stamina is supported by the work of others. They are respected if they have worked hard during their life. There is no respect for the lazy, foolish or dishonest person. (Counts and Counts, 1985).

In the Bible, health, sickness, old age and deaths are seen in relationships to the presence of God, who is the supreme reality and source of all life. God is involved in human life with the sole aim of directing life into salvation in eternity (beyond earthly horizons). The Bible does not provide scientific explanation for suffering, old age and death, but it does give an important role to the old. It is they who help Moses as he is dying. After the flight from Egypt, the Lord announces his covenant to the elders and Moses calls the old adults from the people to relay to them the Word of the Lord (Exodus 19).

When Moses climbs the mountain to receive the tablets of stone, seventy of the Elders of Israel accompany him, as prescribed by the Lord (Exodus 24). Again, the Lord says: 'Assemble seventy elders from Israel, men known to you as elders and officers in the community' (Numbers II Verse 16). The Lord takes the spirit that is upon Moses and confers it on the seventy, who prophesy. Moses rejoins the camp with elders of Israel. (Numbers II verse 30).

St Paul writes in his first letter to Timothy 'Never be harsh with an elder; appeal to him as if he were your father . . . . treat the older women as mothers . .'

In the churches of the Reformation, it is the duty of the elders to oversee discipline and supervise morality. We find that the only difference in Calvinism between pastors and elders is in training and function, rather than rank. There are four types of ministry — pastors, doctors, elders and deacons. The first two teach and preach the Word of God while the deacons help the poor and sick. A committee of twelve elders administer and control the church — these elders hold equal rank with the other ministers.

better life conditions (Brody, 1985; Binstock, 1985). According to official data, disabilities and illnesses increase with age, but it is not known whether the age-specific prevalence of these conditions is changing.

DEMOGRAPHIC DATA

The populations of developed countries are aging. The most important factors in this process are the fertility of past years, a decrease in the number of births after an earlier baby boom and progress in both medical and social care. The variation between continents is indicated in Fig. 2.1. Europe has by far the greatest

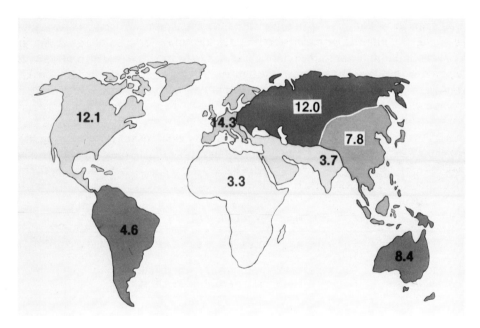

Fig. 2.1   World distribution of population aged over 65 at the end of the present century. *Source*: United Nations. The Old World having a mean value of 14.3% lives up to its name. Africa has the lowest mean age

proportion of elderly people, while the population of the African continent is the youngest (United Nations, 1979). Average life span has recently increased considerably in some countries. For example, in Japan the average span was 76 years for men and 78 years for women in 1969, compared to 42 and 43 between the years 1921 to 1925 (Nakamura, 1982). Icelandic women have the longest average life span of 79 years. In West Germany between 1975 and 1985 the aged population increased by 17% in the age band 75–80, and by 51% and 42% in age bands 80–85 and 85–90. It is calculated that by the year 2000 there will be twice as many people in the world over the age of 80 as there were in 1970. In the last 20 years of this century the number of over-80s will go up by 600,000 in Brazil, 1.3 million in Japan, 2.3 million in India and 5.7 million in China (WHO, 1984).

In Great Britain women make up 51% of the total population (Hodkinson, 1981) and the proportion increases in old age, so that women comprise 58% of those over 65 years old. Beyond 75 years of age the ratio women to men is 2 : 1 and beyond 85 years the same ratio becomes 3 : 1. The increase in the proportion of women among the aged occurs in almost all countries. Women of 65 have an average life expectancy of 16 years compared to 12 years for men. It is calculated that by the turn of the century the difference in favour of females will be about 5.3 years. In the USA the ratio of males to females at birth favours males (105 : 100), but offset against this is the age-dependent mortality index which shows that the death rate is greater in males (Brody, 1984). The reasons for these sex differences are generally unknown, but in other cases specific factors can be identified. For example, the number of males per 1000 females over 75 years of age is 466 in England and Finland with the minimum of 463 in France due to high mortality in the First World War. By contrast, the figure is 914 in Israel, where there has been conspicuous immigration (Grundy and Arie, 1984). The life expectancy among women aged 60 has improved in general by 2.5 years since 1950 but an increase has occurred in men only in Japan (WHO, 1984). The marked reduction in the mortality of older women is therefore the primary cause of sex differences in life expectancy at birth. Table 2.1 indicates differences in male mortality in various

Table 2.1   Mortality among elderly males since 1950 in some countries
(*source*: WHO, 1984)

Reduction:	Japan, France, Spain, Switzerland, Australia, Finland, Poland, USA
Increase:	German Democratic Republic, Netherlands, Norway
Stability:	Denmark, Hungary, Ireland, New Zealand

countries. A number of variables is certainly responsible for the different life expectancies of men and women, including differences in habits (e.g. smoking), exposure to occupational hazards (e.g. mining) and stress (e.g. business). But, in the course of this book we shall frequently find evidence of genetic factors favouring women (see Table 14.3).

In 1900 only a quarter of the population of the USA survived until 65 years of age. By contrast, 70% reaches that age today. Presently, 30% exceeds 80 years of age and the figure is increasing (Brody, 1985). The official statistics report a drop in the American mortality rate. The logarithm of the mortality rate follows a linear function with age. Age-dependent illnesses, such as cancer, vascular diseases, diabetes and dementia, have a similar incidence (Katzman, 1983). In America 1.4 million people reach the age of 65 every 50 weeks. Every day 5000 people reach this milestone and 3600 persons die. Of those remaining, 43% consult their doctor more frequently. More than 75% of that population suffers from chronic and disabling illnesses, such as heart disturbances, arthritis, visual problems and rheumatism (Lewis, 1984). A Swedish study of 365,000 deaths over 5 years found that 46% of husbands die in the first 3 months of widowhood, whereas only 22% of women die in the same period after losing their husband (Mellstrom et al., 1982).

Although life expectancy approaches 90 years, the average human life span does not seem to increase, except perhaps in a few communities with marked endogamy. The areas with the greatest longevity are Vilcabamba in Peru, Hunza in Pakistan, Karabakh in Azerbadijan and Abkhazia in Georgia (Lelashvili and Dalakishvili, 1984). However, caution has to be taken in accepting the data on these super-longevals, because of the poor credibility of local registers (going back to the middle of the last century), difficulty in identifying the subjects and tendency to exaggerate one's own age (Katzman, 1983).

In this century the probability of survival has improved with the age distribution tending toward the well-known 'rectangular' curve. By placing age on the X-axis and the number of survivors on the Y-axis, then in the ideal society, a Shangri-La without pain and troubles, we would have 100% survivors until about 100 years old, followed by a rapid decline. Russian authors have pointed out that in a society such as that of Sweden the age-dependent mortality rate has not changed in the course of the century (Gavrilov et al., 1983). The decline in mortality in the aged is clear. The effect is not entirely due to preventive medicine and other still unknown factors must exist (Brody, 1985). Similar circumstances surround other human changes such as increase in height in successive generations. In the more developed countries, approximately one person out of 10,000 lives beyond 100 years of age (Fries, 1980). In the 21st century Italy will have the satisfaction (if we want to call it that) of leading the world in this classification. Table 2.2 shows that this country with an estimated figure of 16.54% of its people over 65 years of age clearly surpasses even the long-lived Swiss and Swedish. As can be seen from the intercontinental distribution, the countries of the third world take last place with Kenya closing the list at 2.5%. These figures are not equal for the sexes. In Italy's case older men represent 13.85% of the population while older women make up 19.1%, thus confirming the greater longevity of women.

HEALTH AND THE QUALITY OF LIFE IN THE AGED POPULATION

Age is certainly a risk factor for many disabling, neurological illnesses, such as Parkinson's disease, Alzheimer's dementia and cerebral vascular diseases. Fig. 2.2 shows the distribution of admissions in one year, as a function of age in an Italian hospital specializing in rehabilitation. Old women occupy more recovery days in the hospital, in part because once their role of mother, wife and housewife has finished, they are often considered a family burden. The abandonment of the male family head is rarer and motives of honour and respectability should not be overlooked (Fig. 2.3).

The diseases which strike the aged the most are those which affect the

Table 2.2   Percent distribution of the
population over 65 in different countries

Italy	16.4
Sweden	15.8
Switzerland	15.8
West Germany	15.5
England	14.9
Denmark	14.6
Hungary	14.6
Spain	14.6
Japan	14.3
United States	12.2
Canada	11.0
Australia	10.8
China	7.2
Brazil	4.5
India	3.7
Saudi Arabia	3.0
Kenya	2.5

(*source*: United Nations, 1979)

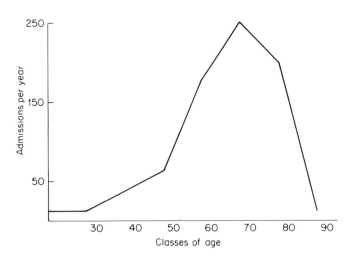

Fig. 2.2   Age distribution of patients in 1985 at S. Giovanni Battista Hospital, one
of the leading centres for rehabilitation in Italy. Age is a risk-factor for stroke

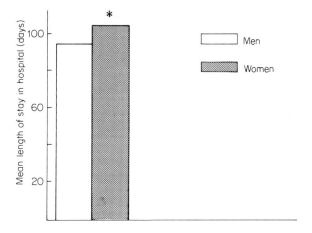

Fig. 2.3 Mean length of stay at S. Giovanni Battista Hospital. Women stay longer than men ($p<0.05$). Year: 1985

cardiovascular system. A multivariate analysis of factors affecting the health of elderly Japanese has revealed a number of biological variables which are inversely related to good health (Benfante et al., 1985). In order of importance, these are age, blood pressure, smoking, obesity, alcohol consumption, serum triglycerides, serum uric acid and serum glucose. On the other hand no relationship was found between state of health and socio-demographic characteristics. From Italian statistical data, 75% of deaths (522,332 in 1982) were of persons over 65 years of age. The causes of death are listed in Table 2.3, from which it is clear that in this country too the circulatory disease is the most important factor.

Table 2.3 Main causes of diseases in a Western country (Italy) on 522,332 cases. Seventy-five percent are patients over 65. Year: 1982

Diseases	%
Circulatory diseases	53.64
Tumours	20.25
Respiratory diseases	7.27
Metabolic, endocrine and immunitary diseases	3.90
Urological diseases	1.65
Neurological diseases	1.17
Infectious and parasitic diseases	0.48

(*source*: National Institute of Statistics, Italy)

It is reasonable to think that the proportion of the aged who are institutionalized bears some relationship with the status and the role of the aged in any given country and that social and economic demographical conditions will also affect these statistics. However, due to the great number of other variables, international comparisons have not demonstrated such effects (Grundy and Arie, 1984). Holland has the highest number of aged in non-private households (10.48 per 1000), while among the countries studied by Grundie and Arie the lowest number belongs to Spain where the figure is 1.90 per 1000. Of people over 65, 4.76 per 1000 are in medical and social welfare institutions in England and 6.55 per 1000 in New Zealand.

The incidence of suicides in the last 10 years has increased in older people (Fig. 2.4), though fortunately (at least in Italy) there has been a drop in suicide

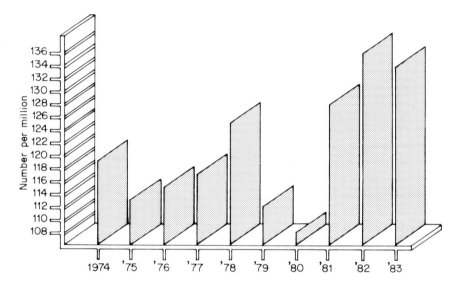

Fig. 2.4 Changing rates of suicide in Italy in the population over 65. A steep increase occurred in recent years, not accounted for by the slight increase in this section of population

among the young. Suicide is 2.5 times more prevalent in men, as Table 2.4 indicates. The interpretation of the figures may indicate on one side a weakening of the historical security in the male and on the other side a greater self-awareness acquired by women. In the decade from 1974–83, the general incidence of suicides was irregular, but the tendency was on the increase in the last 3 years. These figures clearly indicate discomfort, loneliness, loss of interest and motivation and that the meaning of life, which the Japanese call 'ikigai', seems so frequently to be lost (Nakamura, 1982).

The statistics are not uniformly grim; indeed there are hopeful signs. One

Table 2.4 Suicides in a Western country (Italy)
in persons over 65. Distribution by sex

Year	Males	Females
1974	571	227
1975	556	224
1976	583	227
1977	611	237
1978	677	254
1979	251	238
1980	601	242
1981	672	262
1982	728	282
1983	762	279

epidemiological study conducted on more than 2,500 residents in New Haven (Connecticut) over 65 years of age, finds them in a satisfactory condition of well-being. For example, their current 6 month rate of psychiatric disorders is 6.7%, much lower than the percent found in a group of under 45-year-olds in the same community. The percentage of those interviewed who referred to a physical discomfort was 9.9%, while only 3.6% referred to an emotional problem; 73.5% do not have memory problems and only 3.7% request frequent help from friends (Weissman et al., 1985). The American Association of Retired Persons numbers 15 million people in the USA, with their own magazines coming third in national circulation. Unity, as the saying goes, is strength.

Sexual behaviour remains important in old age (see Birren et al., 1983). Sexual activity lessens more in women than men. Widowhood strikes women more often and is thus a limiting factor. There is a gap between interest and sexual activity. Sexual activity may not be tolerated in old people's residences or in nursing homes. Although the frequency of sexual relations diminishes with age, the active sexual life of the aged is surprisingly higher than one would imagine. The youthful drive is substituted by the pleasure enjoyed before and after and the experience may discard taboos and guilt feelings. The physical capacities may lessen but not the pleasure and satisfaction which may be even greater (Renshaw, 1985).

In a study carried out in Italy on 141 females and 159 males aged between 55 and 90, the frequency of sexual activity was found to vary with age. The frequency was high in all groups. Only 10% of the males and 2.6% of the females no longer had sexual relations in the 55–60 years old group, while 34% of the interviewed males over 80 still had occasional sexual intercourse (Fig. 2.5). With respect to the quality of sexual experience, the study showed that only one third of the subjects complained of diminished satisfaction, while 60% enjoyed an actual orgasm. Sexual activity is clearly more frequent in well-to-do persons, males as well as females, but women are more subject to social taboos (Todarello and Boscia, 1985).

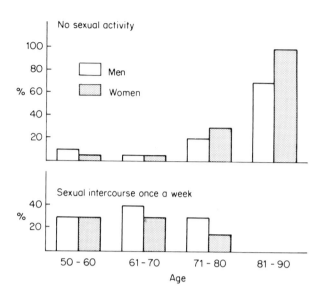

Fig. 2.5 Sexual behaviour among the middle aged and the elderly. The research is based on 141 females and 159 males, between 55 and 90 years of age, in Southern Italy. Adapted from Todarello and Boscia, 1985, with permission

THE FISCAL IMPLICATIONS OF AGING

The economic burden for the state which manages a national health service tends to grow and this is aggravated by the increase in the number of retired people. Epidemiological studies show that the number of the aged with mental disorders, particularly of Alzheimer's type, is increasing in parallel with the general aging. A recent review of studies shows that the incidence of dementia in subjects over 65 years old varies from one country to another with a range 1–9% (Pinessi et al., 1984). If the incidence of dementia among people over 65 were only 2%, in a country like Italy as a whole, the hospitalized demented would occupy a third of the existing bed space.

The successes attained in emergency care and neurosurgery may contribute to elevate the number of demented, restoring life to people with vast brain lesions, such as in strokes, head injuries, cardiac arrest and after brain operations. A new factor may worsen the situation. Care for the demented lengthens their life, even though they may have a shorter life than their peers.

In England the figure is between 5 and 6% (Roth, 1982). In a sample of 499 subjects, 26 demented were identified who then spent 255 weeks in a geriatric institution. In the USA in 1980 there were over 2 million patients affected by Alzheimer's disease with a mean age of 80. It is estimated that in the year 2000 the number will rise to 3.8 million, and continuing in the same trend, to 8.5 million after 50 years. Also in the USA, 1.1 million of the aged are cared for in nursing homes and the number will double by the end of the century (Brody, 1985). The demographic trend called 'the greying of America' raises the problem of expenditure, which in 1983 reached 27% of the annual federal budget, $218 billion on benefits to the aged, and the trend is upward. The main reason is represented by inflation in the cost of health care, which is higher than general inflation in the country (Binstock, 1985).

The increase in the number of the aged causes numerous problems in the areas of health, ethics and society. In a Finnish study, it was observed that 65% of the aged lived in their own homes, 25% in old people's homes and 10% in hospitals in the years 1977–1978. After 5 years the hospitalized group had increased five times, with a rise in cases of dementia, confusion and general problems (Haavisto et al., 1985).

Public expenditure on hospitalization increases and yet hospitalization itself is not the best therapeutic intervention for the aged and demented. What are the valid alternatives in existence today? Can one legitimately refuse an admission in a state-operated hospital which is not strictly necessary? How can a patient not needing hospital care be dismissed, if social services are lacking? Injustices are everywhere in this tangle of problems. On one side, there are the families with their everyday life destroyed by the burden of life with demented relatives, devoid of either minimal home assistance or adequate subsidy. On the other side, there are the aged but not ill, guilty of occupying space at home and therefore hospitalized by their family in geriatric wards. In a welfare system provided by the state, it is not difficult for relatives to force hospital acceptance, where young doctors on duty are intimidated by threats of law suits. Dismissal is anything but easy.

Today one is present at the dawn of the private sector in European medicine, profit-making as opposed to non-profit institutions. Presently, they represent 7% of hospital business in the USA, but according to Wall Street experts, that market will rise 20% in the next 10 years and it is not clear if this will translate into savings (Bulger, 1985). The supporters of the private sector are convinced that savings will be made by reductions in the number of unnecessary hospitalizations and reduction of incompetent staff, which are common in the public services, often imposed by politicians.

There is yet another new social phenomenon: on their retirement, many older competent people are not replaced by a numerically equal population. The entire world, especially European countries have had and still experience very difficult years of recession. Unemployment, youth's lack of motivation, drugs and terrorism are factors where young people have been either victims or perpetrators. For these historical reasons there has been a loss of important aspects of cultural heritage. Worthwhile activities, in agriculture or artisan work for example, have experienced a strong numerical reduction in the work-force and many occupations may disappear altogether. In the last few years, a gap has appeared between the employed and the unemployed. The generation, which in the past always had the chance to work, improved in its own competence, while the generation which for various reasons has had more difficulty finding placements is more inexpert as a consequence. But in many countries in the near future, the 'contented' generation, the ruling class as it were, will have to leave their place of work for reasons of age. Fortunately, many vacancies will be created, but in many of these jobs there is the risk that the former competent person will be replaced by one who is inadequately prepared. Here one poses an important question: can those workers with long experience continue to contribute to their society? Or must they become added burdens to the expenditure of the welfare system, and relegated simply as candidates for dementia, depression and suicide? It is this important issue which makes research into aging and the identification of the meaning of growing old naturally necessary. Either way, the aged will play a major role in the nineties.

Research on the disabling neurological illnesses of old age and above all Alzheimer's dementia still receives insufficient financing. For example, in the USA less than $20 million is spent compared to $1 billion on cancer and cardiocirculatory illnesses (Binstock, 1985). There is a general alert for the need to increase these funds, but there are also polemics concerning their allocation (Holliday, 1984; Davies and Brocklehurst, 1985). Biomedical research concerning chronic illnesses, even though they are highly disabling, is not progressing because it is afflicted by precarious financial resources (Busse, 1985).

REFERENCES

Benfante, R., Reed, D., and Brody, J. (1985). Biological and social predictors of health in an aging cohort. *J. Chron. Dis.*, 18, 385–395.

Benton, A. L., and Sivan, A. B. (1984). Problems and conceptual issues in neuropsychological research in aging and dementia. *J. Clin. Neuropsychol.*, 6, 57–63.

Binstock, R. H. (1985). Health care of the aging: trends, dilemmas, and prospects for the year 2000. In C. M. Gaitz and T. Samorajski (Eds). *Aging 2000: Our Health Care Destiny*. New York: Springer–Verlag, pp. 3–15.

Birren, J. E. (1985). Health care in the 21st century: the social and ethical context. In C. M. Gaitz and T. Samorajski (Eds). *Aging 2000: Our Health Care Destiny*. New York: Springer–Verlag, pp. 521–530.

Birren, J. E., Cunningham, W. R., and Yamamoto, K. (1983). Psychology of adult development and aging. *Ann. Rev. Psychol.*, 34, 543–575.

Brody, J. A. (1984). Facts, projections, and gaps concerning data on aging. *Public Health Rep.*, 99, 468–475.

Brody, J. A. (1985). Prospects for an ageing population. *Nature*, 315, 463–466.

Bulger, R. J. (1985). Old wine in new bottles: medical care for the elderly in the year 2000. In C. M. Gaitz and T. Samorajski (Eds). *Aging 2000: Our Health Care Destiny*. New York: Springer–Verlag, pp. 511–519.

Busse, E. W. (1985). The next twenty years: medical science and the practice of geriatrics. In C. M. Gaitz and T. Samorajski (Eds). *Aging 2000: Our Health Care Destiny*. New York: Springer–Verlag, pp. 17–26.

Côte, L. J., and Kremzner, L. T. (1983). Biochemical changes in normal aging in human brain. In R. Mayeux and W. G. Rosen, *Advances in Neurology*, vol. 38. New York: Raven Press, pp. 19–30.

Davies, J., and Brocklehurst, J. C. (1985). Ageing and research. *Lancet*, 8423, 287–288.

Esposito, J. L. (1983). Conceptual problems in theoretical gerontology. *Perspect. Biol. Med.*, 26, 522–546.

Fries, J. F. (1980). Aging, natural death and the compression of morbidity. *New Engl. J. Med.*, 30, 130–135.

Gavrilov, L. A., Gavrilova, N. S., and Nosov, V. A. (1983). Human life span stopped increasing: why? *Gerontology*, 29, 176–180.

Grundy, E., and Arie, T. (1984). Institutionalization and the elderly: international comparisons. *Age Ageing*, 13, 129–137.

Haavisto, M. V., Heikinheimo, R. J., Mattila, K. J., and Rajala, S. A. (1985). Living conditions and health of a population aged 85 years or over: a five-year follow-up study. *Age Ageing*, 14, 202–208.

Hodkinson, H. M. (1981). *An outline of Geriatrics*. London: Academic Press.

Holliday, R. (1984). The ageing process is a key problem in biomedical research. *Lancet*, 8416, 1386–1387.

Katzman, R. (1983). Overview: demography, definitions and problems. In R. Katzman and R. D. Terry (Eds), *The Neurology of Aging*. Philadelphia: F. A. Davis Co., pp. 1–14.

Lelashvili, N. G., and Dalakishvili, S. M. (1984). Genetic study of high longevity index populations. *Mech. Aging Dev.*, 28, 261–271.

Lewis, C. B. (1984). Rehabilitation of the older person: a psychosocial focus. *Phys. Ther.*, 64, 517–522.

Markides, K. S., Timbers, D. M., and Osberg, J. S. (1984). Aging and health: a longitudinal study. *Arch. Gerontol. Geriat.*, 3, 33–49.

Mellstrom, D., Nilsson, A., Oden, A., Rundren, A., and Svanborg, A. (1982). Mortality among the widowed in Sweden. *Scand. J. Soc. Med.*, 10, 33–41.

Nakamura, S. (1982). Anthropological, behavioral and psychosocial factors in neuronal aging. In R. D. Terry, C. L. Bolis and G. Toffano (Eds), *Aging*, vol. 18. New York: Raven Press, pp. 197–207.

Neugarten, B. L. (1984). Psychological aspects of aging and illness. *Psychosomatics*, 25, 123–125.

Pinessi, L., Rainero, I., Asteggiano, G., Ferrero, P., Tarenzi, L., and Bergamasco, B. (1984). Primary dementias: epidemiologic and sociomedical aspects. *Ital. J. Neurol. Sci.*, 5, 51–55.

Renshaw, D. C. (1985). Sex, age, and values *J. Amer. Geriat. Soc.*, 33, 635–643.

Roth, M. (1982). Dementia in relation to aging in the central nervous system. In R. D. Terry, C. L. Bolis and G. Toffano (Eds), *Aging*, vol. 18. New York: Raven Press, pp. 231–250.

Todarello, O., and Boscia, F. M. (1985). Sexuality in the aged: a study of a group of 300 elderly men and women. *J. Endocrinol. Invest.* 8 (suppl. 2), 123–130.

United Nations, Dept. Intern. Econ. Social Affairs (1979). *World population trends and prospect by country*: 1950–2000.

Weissman, M. M., Myers, J. K., Tischler, G. L., Holzer III, C. E., Leaf, P. J., Orvaschel, H., and Brody, J. A. (1985). Psychiatric disorders (DSM-III) and cognitive impairment among the elderly in a U.S. urban community. *Acta Psychiat. Scand.*, 71, 366–379.

World Health Organization (1984). The uses of the epidemiology in the study of the elderly. *Technical Report Series* 706. Geneva, WHO.

CHAPTER 3

Biology and genetics of cellular aging

Is there any support for the contention that if you want a long life, you must choose long-lived parents?

What is biological aging? As of today there is no consensus among biologists on an operational definition of aging. If we accept the premise that aging is a genetically programmed process, when does it start? Is the embryonic development which results in the differentiation of tissues a specialized form of aging? If so the aging process could consist of two phases. The first may be regarded as one of evolution while the second phase may be seen as involution. Commonly the term aging refers only to the second phase. To differentiate the second phase from the first, the term senescence is often used. We will use both words — aging and senescence — to denote the later phase only. To avoid any controversy, we can safely define biological aging as a process involving normal, inherent and progressive change of biological function over the life span. Any definition of aging or explanation of its biological control should encompass two important features: 1) The adaptability of an organism to its normal environment gradually declines following the onset of maturity. We shall deal with the various types of behavioural decline associated to human aging in later chapters. 2) The life span of each species is specified. For example, a mouse lives for about 2.5 years and a man lives for about 80 years. For an understanding of these features we must first turn to biology and genetics.

Table 3.2   Some theories on aging

Wear and tear	A continuous breakdown in cells and organs
Cross-linking	A binding of cell molecules
Clinker	Accumulation of deleterious by-products
Error-catastrophe	Various events change the nucleotide sequence
Mistranscription	The two strands of the DNA double helix become stiffer
Mistranslation	The mRNA template is defective
Program	Aging genes regulate the aging process
Dysdifferentiation	A drifting away of cells from their differentiation
Membrane thickness	Lipid peroxidation impairs transbilayer asymmetry.

asymmetry of the lipid layers in the cell membrane and abolishes transmembrane fluidity differences, thus leading to an impairment of the cell function (Schroeder, 1984).

GENE REGULATION OF AGING

The most attractive explanation of the phenomena of aging is offered by the 'gene regulation theory' of aging, which proposes that the mechanism of aging is analogous to that of normal differentiation and growth. This model is intriguing because it offers an explanation for the two important features of aging discussed earlier, the gradual decline in the activity of an organism after maturity and the specified life span of species. In this context we would recapitulate here the main features of the biological control of eucaryotic gene action during normal development. The gene regulation theory of cellular differentiation is widely accepted. According to this theory, cell specialization occurs by the sequential expression of different genes. One of the earliest pieces of experimental evidence was the sequential activation and inactivation of various genes located in different chromosomes of an insect larva during the course of differentiation. The synthesis of the various polypeptide chains of haemoglobin which is under the control of separate genes of an organism offers a more sophisticated and well-studied example of such sequential gene expression. The epsilon, gamma and beta genes of haemoglobin become active in that order during the early development period. The period when each gene remains active is different and depends on the physiology of the developing individual.

The maximum life span and the average life span of various species seem to be regulated genetically. Table 3.3 lists the life span of some mammals as compiled by Kanungo (1975). The idea that with aging every system malfunctions is not valid. Some enzyme levels indeed decrease and some remain unchanged, but levels of yet other enzymes increase with age (Moudgil and Kanungo, 1973).

Beginning with these general observations we can now examine how the gene regulation theory explains the two important features of aging.

Table 3.3   Life span of some animals

Animals	Longevity (months)	Animals	Longevity (months)
Man	1200	Dog	240
Elephant	780	Cow	180
Horse	660	Fox	174
Mule	576	Rabbit	130
Hippopotamus	540	Guinea-pig	90
Black bear	408	White rat	42
Domestic cat	372	Laboratory mouse	30
Baboon	342	Golden hamster	30
Camel	300		

Functional deterioration of the organism following maturity

Procreation is the prime necessity of the species. New individuals more adaptive to environment arise by procreation. It follows that individuals with higher reproductive capacity persist due to their beneficial nature to the species and their greater selection potential. However, continuous reproduction in an individual would deplete it of certain essential adaptive factors and might lead to its weakness. The law of natural selection has two choices. Either it should develop a process by which the depleted factors of the individual are replenished or the individual is eliminated by death from the population, so that young animals having higher potential can reproduce. Thus, the process of sequential gene activation and repression so well adopted evolutionarily in differentiation and development might continue to eliminate individuals after the reproductive years for the benefit of the species.

Determination of the life span

In any species, each phase of its life span such as differentiation, growth, maturity and senescence has its own duration, speed and mechanisms of control. This is guided by a complex set of regulatory processes with a fixed time course. Certain drastic changes in this regulatory mechanism might lead to shortened life span or death and elimination of the individual. Barring accidents normal genetic functioning will therefore lead to a life of standard duration.

CELLULAR CHANGES ACCOMPANYING AGING

Cell growth

In the early 1960s Hayflick reported that human embryonic fibroblast cells cultured in vitro undergo only a finite number of divisions and then die (1961, 1965, 1984). After a vigorous proliferation, these cells show a gradual slowing of cell division resulting in their ultimate degeneration. These experiments might indicate that death is an intrinsic property of the cell. The cell doubling time of 50

±10 passages, as estimated for human embryonic diploid fibroblast by Hayflick, is rather rigidly respected by the cells. For instance, cells frozen at any passage upon thawing and reculturing, could grow only for the remaining number of passages. Yet some cells, e.g. certain lines of mouse fibroblasts, display indefinite multiplications, due to spontaneous transformation and hence cannot be accepted as normal. Diploid cells in culture offer an ideal experimental model to study the aging phenomenon at cellular level, because the structural and functional alteration identified in the cells could be easily correlated to the number of divisions undergone by the cells. More important, the finite number of cell divisions in vitro, outside the complex regulatory process of the organism confirms the encoding of the life span at the genomic level. This further supports the gene regulation theory of aging.

Biochemical changes

When a cell ages, a series of morphological and physiochemical changes take place. Some of the pertinent changes occurring at the cellular level are enumerated in Table 3.4. A careful study of the literature would reveal that many other

Table 3.4   Morphological and physiochemical changes in the cell

1) Accumulation of the 'exhaustion' pigment ('wear and tear' pigments) are observed particularly in the nerve cells and in the myocardial tissue. This pigment is derived from oxidation of unsaturated lipids. (The accumulation of these pigments is due to the progressive difficulty the cells have in excreting poorly soluble products)
2) Accumulation of small lipid droplets
3) Decrease of cell volume (hypotrophy)
4) Increase in the calcium content of blood and several other tissues and peripheral zone of the cells
5) Increase in iron and potassium
6) Decrease in magnesium
7) Increase in cholesterol and insoluble proteins like globulins
8) Decrease of several enzymatic systems like acid and alkaline phosphatases and esterases
9) Decrease of tissue respiration
10) Inhibition of protein synthesis
11) The increase in covalent cross-linkings in collagen (the solubility of this molecule is reduced, for example, the lens in the eye becomes harder and harder with age due to increased –S–S linkage)
12) Peroxidase damage to membrane lipids appears to impair the transbilayer distribution of phospholipids and possibly cholesterol.

changes accompanying aging might be added to the list. Remarkably, as we shall see later, all these biological changes take place without evident deterioration in the behaviour of normal elderly people as revealed by neurophysiological and neuropsychological examination.

Structural changes in the genome

The genetic material of the eukaryotic cell is organized into chromosomes containing the core DNA, the hereditary principle of the cell, which is surrounded by various types of basic and acidic proteins and some low molecular weight RNAs known as chromosomal RNAs. Indeed during cell division the daughter cells receive a completely organized chromosomal set with, probably, all the associated proteins. The nucleoprotein fibres of which the chromosomes are composed are termed chromatin.

Several structural changes at the level of chromosomes take place in aged cells. Some of anomalies recorded in human lymphocyte chromosomes include chromosomal breaks, chromatid exchange and fragmentation (Dutkowski et al., 1985). Sister chromatid exchanges (SCE) result from chromosomal instability encountered in some diseased conditions, but can also be induced by exposing the cells to nucleotide analogues such as 5-bromo-deoxyuridine. As mentioned earlier, nucleotide analogues also induce aging in cultured cells. Loss of certain specific parts of chromosomes such as centromeres or even entire chromosomes have been widely reported (Jacobs et al., 1964; Nakagome et al., 1984). These augmented structural alterations support the hypothesis that chromosomal instability increases with age.

Changes in chromatin

The fine structure of chromatin has been the subject of detailed investigations in recent years in the hope of understanding the molecular mechanism of differential gene expression during development, differentiation and neoplasia. In brief, the double helical DNA is supercoiled and in the grooves of the supercoils it accomodates different types of basic and acidic proteins. The basic proteins called histones render the chromatin a bead-like nucleosomal structure, by giving a three-dimensional configuration to the DNA helix. The various types of acid proteins associated with chromatin form the major component of the chromosomal proteins and seem to be responsible for tuning DNA replication and RNA transcription. Several types of low molecular weight RNAs are variously associated with the chromosomes and are often claimed to have important roles in gene regulation, though there is no definite experimental evidence for this.

Changes in chromosomal proteins

In evolutionary terms, histones are among the most stable proteins. Hence, it is reasonable to suppose that the major types of histone change very little during aging. In general, a constant DNA:histone ratio is recorded during the mammalian life span (Kanungo, 1980; Medvedev, 1981). This finding is consistent with the observation of unchanged basic nucleosome structure during aging. However, the highly variable H1° histone does increase during mammalian aging (Medvedev et al. 1977 and 1978; Wagner et al. 1982). In addition there are marked changes in the post synthetic modifications, such as increased methylation and decreased phosphorylation and acetylation of histones in aging tissues.

These modifications are closely related to nucleosome structural modulations and hence gene expression. Non-histone proteins (NHP) have a major and more active role in gene regulation (Cartwright et al., 1982) and their pattern is tissue specific. Thus, studies in NHP might offer more insight into the understanding of molecular aging. Two liver-specific NHPs, discovered in rat by Medvedev's group, show an apparent age-related increase (for review see Medvedev, 1984). Furthermore, an age-related decrease of phosphorylation and acetylation of NHPs has been reported in rat brain (Bose and Kanungo, 1982). Distribution of NHP proteins in different parts of the chromatin differs greatly both in quantity and quality. The active part of the chromatin called euchromatin is enriched by NHP, whereas the heterochromatin — the inactive portion of the chromatin is depleted of NHP. Determination of age-related changes in NHP indicated a distinct increase of these proteins in the active chromatin of the rat liver and intestinal mucosa and the same NHPs are usually absent in the inactive heterochromatin. This might explain the general decline of transcription and template activity in the older cells.

Differences in the DNA sequences

The concept that the primary sequences of the genomic DNA of different cells of a given organism is the same has become outdated. In recent years several alterations, both at the level of DNA polymerization as well as post-replicative modifications, have been widely reported and have become the candidates for the mechanism of differential gene expression.

DNA modification and cellular aging

Three types of DNA modification have received attention in recent years. One is a structural modification of the one-dimensional message by the insertion of transposable (mobile) genetic elements. Another is a base modification by methylation, which might change the affinity for other molecules such as proteins, and thereby might alter transcriptional properties of particular genes. The third is a newly discovered three-dimensional structural form, called Z-DNA, which is related to the base sequence, the modification by methylation, the three-dimensional properties and the molecular environment as such. We shall devote the discussion here primarily to DNA modification by methylation, because more is known about this point than the others with respect to aging. The cytosine of the eucaryotic DNA is post-replicatively methylated by an enzyme, DNA-methyltransferase, at certain sites of the genome and this methylation process was suggested to have an important role in cell differentiation and development. In recent years, it has been demonstrated that specific demethylation at crucial sites of the genome would lead to the activation of functional genes and could also induce differentiation (McGhee and Ginder, 1979; Maharajan et al., 1986; De Petrocellis et al., 1986). The earliest indications of age dependent variation in

DNA methylation was reported in the Pacific salmon. It has also been noticed that the 5-methyl-cytosine (mC) content decreases during aging in many mammals (Vanyushin et al., 1973). Thus, in early embryos the mC content is high and decreases sharply soon after birth. In some tissues (brain and heart muscles) it continues to decrease by 30–40% with age. Although in vitro studies have revealed that DNA from aged tissue is potentially capable of being methylated, the reason for the normally low level of methylation in aged organs might be a decreased methyltransferase activity. In any case, a decline in DNA methylation may somehow be responsible for the defective DNA replication and transcription in aged cells.

DNA repair synthesis and ageing

During its life span an organism is exposed to several evironmental agents having DNA damaging effects. Even within the cellular milieu enzymes capable of damaging DNA (excision enzymes) are abundant. The genetic material over-comes this inherent problem by an ingenious process called DNA repair synthesis. Such repair processes, depending on the type of breaks in the DNA, are excision repair, or single or double strand repair. These repair processes are catalysed by specific enzymes called repairases. The potential to repair damage in the DNA could be considered as a safety mechanism to avoid genetic malfunctions of the cells. Several authors claim correlation between cellular aging and alterations in the integrity of DNA structure, such as strand breaks (for review see Nieder-mueller, 1982). Also it is widely claimed that the aging process is characterized by decreased ability to repair damages in DNA (Williams, 1976). Hence a linear relationship between the life span of a species and its potential to repair the DNA has been claimed (Hart and Setlow, 1974). This is sustained by the evidence that genetic diseases of premature aging, such as progeria syndrome, are characterized by lowered efficiency for DNA repair. Mouse fibroblasts in vitro revealed decreased repair synthesis as a function of the donor's age (Kempf et al., 1984). However, the same authors have demonstrated differences in repair synthesis between individuals of a given age group. Studies using human epidermal cells also have failed to confirm a strict relation between aging and DNA repair synthesis (Nette et al., 1984). More recent and detailed studies have indicated: 1) the existence of distinct age-dependent excision repair, 2) a reduction of single-strand breaks, but 3) no significant change in double strand repair as a function of age. Thus, during different stages of life different mechanisms of DNA repair seem to operate (Niedermuller et al., 1985). Does this mean that different types of DNA damage occur preferentially at different phases of the life cycle?

Role of non-genomic DNA in aging

Transfer of mitochondrial DNA sequences to the nucleus has occurred in the course of evolution (Farelly and Buton, 1983; Van den Boogart et al., 1982) and it has been suggested that this transfer was involved in the appearance and growth of tumours. On the basis of hybridization experiments, the occurrence of transposition and amplification of some mitochondrial DNA in *Podospora anserina* nucleus was reported (Wright and Cummings, 1983). Since this amplification was associated with senescence, it was suggested that the transposition of mitochondrial DNA to the nuclear genome and its amplification might cause senescence. Pereira-Smith et al. (1985) have found the senescent cells to produce a membrane-associated protein that inhibits DNA synthesis at the strand replication level. They have also identified a species of mRNA having growth inhibitory effect. This poly A+ mRNA is present in a very high concentration (0.8% of the total mRNA) in senescent human fibroblasts whereas in serum deprived quiescent cells it is only present at 0.005%. However, the coding potential of this mRNA(s) has not yet been investigated (Lumpkin et al., 1986).

Role of immunogenetics in aging

The deficiencies associated with immunological functions have not been proved to be fundamental in the aetiology of age-associated diseases, such as autoimmunity and the degeneration of vascular, renal and central nervous systems. The innumerable age-associated diseases and related physiological changes are due, at least in part, to changes in immune functions. Two important factors in immune dysfunctions associated with the pathogenesis of aging are the thymic clock and the major histocompatibility complex (MHC) associated control of immune response and resistance to diseases. The MHC controls antigen recognition, antibody production, lymphocyte proliferation and the suppression of the immune response. The possible role of the immune system in aging was first proposed by Walford (1969) and was further developed by Burnet (1971). This hypothesis was supported by the early evidence that the decline in the immune capacity of old age is related to similar diseases arising in T-cell deficient mammals (Good and Yunis, 1974). It is possible that thymic involution has an important bearing on aging and that the former is genetically controlled. For instance, the differentiation of thymocytes might cease due to changes in the endocrine centres of the central nervous system (CNS). Since T-cells are known to control the B-lymphocyte development, a shift in CNS endocrine controls might cause decline in both humoral as well as in cell mediated immunity. A large body of evidence exists to support this concept (Siegel and Good, 1972).

REFERENCES

Alexander, P. (1967). Genetic changes in aging. In P. Alexander (Ed.), *Aspects of the Biology of Aging*. Cambridge: Cambridge University Press, pp. 29–52.
Bose, R., and Kanungo, M. S. (1982). Polyamines modulate phosphorylation and acetylation of non-histone chromosomal proteins of the cerebral cortex of rats of various ages. *Arch. Gerontol. Geriat.*, 1, 339–348.
Burnet, F. M. (1971). An immunological approach to aging. *Lancet*, ii, 358–360.
Cartwright, I. L., Abmayr, S. M., Fleischmann, G., Lowenhaupt, K., Elgin, S. C. R., Keene, M. A., and Howard, G. C. (1982). The role of nonhistone chromosomal proteins. *CRC Crit. Rev. Biochem.*, 13, 1–86.
De Petrocellis, L., Maharajan, V., De Petrocellis, B., and Minei, R. (1986). Bud induction

in decapitated *Hydra attenuata* by 5-azacytidine: a morphological study. *J. Emb. Exp. Morphol.*, 93, 105–119.

Dutkowski, R. T., Lesh, R., Staiano-Coco, L., Thaler, H., Darlington, G. J., and Weksler, M. E. (1985). Increased chromosomal instability in lymphocytes for elderly humans. *Mutation Res.*, 149, 505–512.

Farelly, F., and Buton, R. A. (1983). Rearranged mitochondrial genes in the yeast nuclear genome. *Nature*, 301, 296–301.

Good, R. A., and Yunis, E. J. (1974). Association of autoimmunity, immunodeficiency and aging in man, rabbits and mice. *Fed. Proc.*, 33, 2040–2050.

Hart, R. W., and Setlow, R. B. (1974). Correlation between deoxyribonucleic acid excision-repair and life-span in a number of mammalian species. *Proc. Natl. Acad. Sci. U.S.A.*, 71, 2169–2173.

Hayflick, L. (1965). The limited in vitro lifetime of human diploid cell strains. *Exp. Cell Res.* 37, 614–636.

Hayflick, L. (1984). Intracellular determinants of cell aging. *Mech. Ageing Dev.*, 28, 177–185.

Hayflick, L., and Moorhead, P. S. (1961). The serial cultivation of human diploid cell strains. *Exp. Cell Res.*, 25, 585–621.

Holliday, R., and Tarrant, G. M. (1972). Altered enzymes in ageing human fibroblasts. *Nature*, 238, 26–30.

Jacobs, P. A., Brunton, M., and Court Brown, W. M. (1964). Cytogenetic studies in leucocytes on the general population; subjects by ages 65 years and more. *Am. Hum. Genet.* 27, 353–365.

Kanungo, M. S. (1975). A model for ageing. *J. Theor. Biol.*, 53, 253–261.

Kanungo, M. S. (1980). *Biochemistry of Aging.* Academic Press, New York.

Kempf, C., Schmitt, M., Danse, J. M., and Kempf, J. (1984). Correlation of DNA repair synthesis with ageing in mice, evidenced by quantitative autoradiography. *Mech. Ageing Dev.*, 26, 183–194.

Lumpkin, C. K., jr., McClung, J. K., Pereira-Smith, O. M., and Smith, J. R. (1986). Existence of high abundance antiproliferative mRNA's in senescent human diploid fibroblasts. *Science*, 232, 393–395.

Maharajan, P., Maharajan, V., Branno, E., and Scarano, E. (1986). Effects of 5-azacytidine on DNA methylation and early development of sea urchins and ascidia. *Differentiation*, 32, 200–207.

McGhee, J. D., and Ginder, G. D. (1979). Specific DNA methylation sites in the vicinity of the chicken beta-globin genes. *Nature*, 280, 419–420.

Medvedev, Z. A. (1981). Chromatin proteins and cellular ageing. In J. W. Rohen (Ed.), *Biomedical and Morphological Aspects of Ageing.* Wiesbaden: Steiner Verlag, pp. 125–148.

Medvedev, Z. A. (1984). Age changes of chromatin. A review. *Mech. Ageing Dev.*, 28, 139–154.

Medvedev, Z. A., Medvedeva, M. N., and Huschcha (1977). Age changes of the pattern of F1 histone subfractions in rat liver and spleen chromatin. *Gerontology*, 23, 334–341.

Medvedev, Z. A., Medvedeva, M. N., and Robson, L. (1978). Tissue specificity and age changes of the pattern of the H1 group of histones in chromatin from mouse tissue. *Gerontology*, 24, 286–292.

Moudgil, V. K., and Kanungo, M. S. (1973). Effect of age of the rat on induction of acetylcholinesterase of the brain by 17-beta-estradiol. *Biochim. Biophys. Acta*, 329, 211–220.

Nakagome, Y., Abe, T., Misawa, S., Takeshita, T., and Iinuma, K. (1984). The loss of centromeres from chromosomes of aged women. *Am. J. Hum. Genet.*, 36, 398–404.

Nette, E. G., Xi, Y. P., Sun, Y. K., Andrews, A. D., and King, D. W. (1984). A correlation between aging and DNA repair in human epidermal cells. *Mech. Ageing Dev.*, 24, 283–292.

Niedermueller, H. (1982). Age dependency of DNA repair in rats after DNA damage by carcinogens. *Mech. Ageing Res.*, 19, 259.

Niedermueller, H., Hofecker, G., and Skalicky, M. (1985). Changes of DNA repair mechanisms during the ageing of the rat. *Mech. Ageing Dev.*, 29, 221–238.

Orgel, L. E. (1973). Aging of clones of mammalian cells. *Nature*, 243, 441–445.

Pereira-Smith, O. M., Fisher, S. F., and Smith, J. R. (1985). Senescent and quiescent cell inhibitors of DNA synthesis membrane-associated proteins. *Exp. Cell Res.*, 160, 297–306.

Reis, S. U., and Rothstein, M. (1974). Age-related change in specific activity of isocitrate lyase from turbatrix aceti. *Fed. Proc.*, 33, 1308.

Schroeder, F. (1984). Role of membrane lipid asymmetry in aging. *Neurobiology of Aging*, 5, 323–333.

Seegmiller, J. E. (1985). Molecular biology of aging. Gene stability and gene expression. In R. S. Sohal, L. Birnbaum and R. G. Cutler (Eds), *Aging*, vol. 29, New York: Raven Press, pp. 1–6.

Siegel, M., and Good, R. A. (1972). *Tolerance, Autoimmunity and Ageing*. Springfield: Thomas.

Strehler, B. L., Hirsh, G., Gusseck, D., Johnson, R., and Bick, M. (1971). Codon-restriction theory in aging and development. *J. Theor. Biol.*, 33, 429–474.

Van den Boogaart, P., Samallo, J., and Agsteribbe, E. (1982). Similar genes for a mitochondrial ATPase subunit in the nuclear and mitochondrial genomes of Neurospora. *Nature*, 298, 187–189.

Vanyushin, B. F., Nemirovski, L. E., Klimengo, V. V., Vasilyev, V. K., and Belozersky, A. N. (1973). The 5-Methylcytosine in DNA of rats. *Gerontologia*, 19, 138–152.

Wagner, A. P., Iordachel, M. C., and Wagner, L. P. (1982). Age changes in the H1 group of histones from rat liver. *Exp. Gerontol.*, 17, 173–177.

Walford, R. L. (1969). *The immunological Theory of Ageing*. Copenhagen: Munskgaard.

Williams, J. R. (1976). Role of DNA repair in cell inactivation, aging and transformation: a selective review, a speculative model. *Adv. Radiat. Biol.*, 6, 161.

Wright, R. M., and Cummings, D. J. (1983). Integration of mitochondrial gene sequences within the nuclear genome during senescence in a fungus. *Nature*, 302, 86–88.

Zeelon, P., Gershon, H., and Gershon, D. (1973). Inactive enzyme molecules in aging organism. Nematode fructose-1,6 diphosphate aldolase. *Biochemistry*, 12, 1743–1750.

CHAPTER 4

The histological drama

The aging brain loses weight, volume, neurons. It acquires histological features which also occur in Alzheimer's disease. What is the relationship between aging and dementia?

The problem of aging has promoted intensive histological investigation aimed at identifying the changes which take place in the cellular structure of the brain. As we shall see, the histological appearance of both grey and white matter is profoundly altered throughout the aging nervous system. However, somewhat similar changes are found in dementia so that it is not yet possible to make any clear distinction between the normal process of aging and the pathological features of Alzheimer's disease.

Before we look at the findings in detail it is important to draw attention to the problems involved in carrying out such studies and interpreting the data, problems which may obscure both age related changes and any distinguishing features of dementia.

First of all, there are technical difficulties surrounding the collection and processing of post mortem brain tissue. Autolytic changes take place in the period between death and the collection and freezing of specimens of brain tissue. Further changes take place during the freezing process itself and during storage. Such degradation of the tissue may obscure significant structural features. The illness which preceded death may have brought about its own changes in nervous tissue which then become confounded with those of aging. Both of these problems can be avoided to some extent in laboratory experiments on animals. The difficulty with animal studies is that we do not know whether they adequately model the alterations which take place in human senility.

The literature on the histopathology of aging has accumulated over many years. Until recently the large majority of studies had not been supported with adequate details of the population sample and terminal diagnoses, particularly with regard to the distinction between aging and dementia. It is often impossible to recover this information a posteriori, indeed many of the diagnostic tests which provide accurate information today were not available when the studies were carried out. We shall see just how important accurate classification is when we deal with investigations using electroencephalography, evoked potentials and Positron Emission Tomography. In histopathology there are relatively few recent studies of normal aging. Many papers and monographs which purport to deal with the subject in fact concentrate on Alzheimer's disease. We are therefore obliged to draw much of our information from old data in which the changes in dementia and aging may be confounded.

With these caveats in mind, we must nevertheless proceed. The major changes which have been associated with aging and Alzheimer's disease are listed in Table 4.1.

Table 4.1   Main morphological changes in the aging brain

1) decrease of brain weight
2) decrease of brain volume
3) variations in neurons and glia
4) dendritic loss
5) widening of sulci and ventricles
6) senile plaques
7) tangles
8) deposit of lipofuscin
9) capillary alterations
10) deposit of aluminium
11) deposit of copper
12) deposit of iron
13) deposit of melanin

The weight of the brain reaches its peak at the age of 25. On the average it weighs 1400 g in men and 1260 g in women. Famous historical examples rule out a relationship between weight and mental ability. There is strong agreement about the loss of weight in the old brain. A decrease of about 10% has been reported

(Brody, 1955; Blinkov and Glezer, 1968; Brody, 1973; Dekaban and Sadowski, 1978). So-called cohort effects tend to overestimate the loss in the old group (Corsellis, 1976): during the first fifty years of life, grey matter is lost at a greater rate than white, whereas in the second fifty years the loss in the white matter is relatively higher.

Apparently, the loss is not very different from that shown by demented subjects. Autopsy findings in 14 patients affected by Alzheimer's dementia compared with measurements on 10 normal age-matched subjects, indicate that the mean weight of the Alzheimer's brains can be only 8% less than that of the normals (Terry, 1982). Neuropathological studies on three groups of subjects (normal middle-aged, normal elderly and senile dementia) show that the weight loss in both elderly groups is similar, namely 17% compared to the middle-age group (DeKosky and Bass, 1980). The normal subjects died from either accidental trauma or acute cardiac arrest, thus offsetting a bias due to disease-induced brain alterations. In parallel with the weight loss, there is an age-dependent volume loss. The advent of the CT-scan era has provided non-invasive proof of the autopsy and pneumoencephalographic findings of brain shrinkage with age. Sulci and ventricular spaces are wider after the age of 40 as we shall see in Chapter 6. The ability to separate the brains of elderly and demented subjects by means of CT-scan is still unproven. On the other hand, at least 50 and generally 100 ml of brain parenchyma must be lost before clinical multi-infarct dementia is recognizable (Tomlinson et al., 1970). In some cases of Alzheimer's dementia there is a huge atrophy, whereas other cases are apparently not too different from age-matched normal controls. Such contradictory findings may lead us to conflicting conclusions and it is therefore unsafe to place much value on gross anatomical findings. In Chapter 6 data on the lack of precise correlations between CT-scan and neuropsychological performance will be discussed further. In the elderly brain alterations occur in the grey matter as well as in the white. Perhaps, in the late decades, large neurons die off and large myelinated axons degenerate in their track within the white matter (Terry, 1980).

There is no doubt about the correlation between weight and neuronal loss. The precise values vary somewhat, since some calculations include the basal ganglia, brain stem and cerebellum and others do not. Some counts hypothesize 100 billion neurons, waning at the rate of 100,000 per day; this decay would lead to a 19.7% reduction at the age of 80 years (Meier-Ruge et al., 1978). Phylogenetic neuronal loss seems to be higher in the heaviest brains like the human one, suggesting that the aging process is not the same for all species. However, both small neurons (Brody, 1955 and 1973; DeKosky and Bass, 1980) and large neurons (Henderson et al., 1980) are affected.

A recent study carried out on three groups (old-old, 85–94 years; elderly, 65–74; young controls) demonstrated a lack of differences between elderly and young controls. By contrast, smaller cell bodies characterize the old-old group, especially in the external pyramidal layer (Schulz and Hunzinger, 1980). Many synaptic connections of each neuron are lost, not only at telencephalic level, but also in the cerebellum, where a 25% loss may take place in a 100-year age span. The effect is not appreciable until the sixth decade of life (see Gilloteaux and Linz,

1984, for review). Russian researchers found a decrease in the quantity of axosomatic and axodendritic synapses in motor and visual areas with thinning of synaptic membranes, shortening of synaptic contacts and a reduced number of synaptic vesicles (Artukhina quoted by Orlovskaya, 1982). Again, the cellular count gives similar results in both elderly and demented patients (Tomlinson et al., 1970; DeKosky and Bass, 1980; Terry, 1980 and 1982). Supporters of the theory 'dementia=exaggerated aging' base their arguments on observations like these.

Some cerebral areas seem to be especially vulnerable. Neuronal loss has been found in the superior temporal gyrus (Brody, 1955), while other structures seem to be spared, for example some nuclei in the brain stem (Konigsmark and Murphy, 1970; Monagle and Brody, 1974). According to researchers of the Lubeck group (Haug et al., 1983) each part of the brain has its own part in the aging process. Some cortical areas are resistant, e.g. areas 7 and 17 (parietal and occipital cortex), whereas some others undergo a 15% shrinkage, e.g. areas 6 and 11 (extrapyramidal and orbital cortex). These data are confirmed by another investigation in which slight differences are also observed between elderly and demented patients. Using an automatic cell counting technique on nine brain areas, relatively smaller neuronal population is seen in frontal and superior temporal areas in Alzheimer's dementia. The same is not true of parietal and occipital sites (Mountjoy et al., 1983). The frontal but not the temporal cortex shows a statistically significant decrease with age in the number of synapses, which were counted in columns of neuropil oriented at right angles to the pia (Gibson, 1983).

Subcortical structures, such as the corpus striatum and dentate nucleus, undergo a parallel cell loss with age. These grey structures are reduced in relation to the hemispheres without sex differences or asymmetries (Murphy, 1985), a process which affects left and right hemispheres and males and females equally. The loss begins at puberty and its time course varies from structure to structure. Cell loss also takes place in the putamen, where small and large cells are equally affected (Bugiani et al., 1978).

Relatively little is known of the age dependent changes in dendritic fields. It appears that neurons undergo subtle alterations with progressive loss of the horizontally oriented dendritic system in areas that are known to receive specific synaptic terminals from intracortical fibre systems. The intertwined and bundled network is proposed as storage sites for central processing (Scheibel and Scheibel, 1975). The loss of dendritic arborization and the cellular decrease are supposed to damage the computing capabilities of the nervous tissue along with mismanagement of coded outputs. The highest variations take place in the third cortical layer, where the thick interconnections with short-axon cells may have a bearing on the process of memory storage. These cortical changes have recently been confirmed in a layer-by-layer EM study (Iontov, 1984). Alterations are found in the cytoplasm, neurocytes, dendrites, spines, axons and their terminals and are likewise interpreted as the histopathological basis of forgetfulness in the elderly. However, there is some disagreement as to the cortical layers most affected. According to some observations (Nakamura et al., 1985) basal dendrites of the pyramidal cells decrease in number with age and the layer V is especially affected. In Chapter 8, we shall present a tentative explanation for central slowing with age, by considering the defective exchange of information among the dendrites of these cells. Since the EEG is produced by the activity of a large number of vertical loops in the superficial cortical layers, which sweep across the cortical surface, dendritic variations should produce EEG variations. Accordingly, we shall consider age-dependent EEG changes in Chapter 7. Whatever histopathological changes are eventually found among the dendrites, it seems likely that the nature and speed of the damage will prove more important than its extent for this will affect the capacity of the system to adapt to the effects of the changes.

The amount of myelin in the stria of Gennari in the human striate cortex undergoes a natural reduction with advancing age (Lintl and Braak, 1983). The fibre population in the human optic nerve is also affected. There is a loss of 400,000 fibres over a 70-year life span, with an estimated loss of around 5,600 axons per year; a 70-year-old subject may be expected to have 1,250,000 nerve fibres in the optic nerve (Balaszi et al., 1984). Although neurons and glial cells are both affected by aging processes, it is not yet clear how the extent of the loss compares in Alzheimer's disease.

Histological studies indicate merely a quantitative difference (Tomlinson and Henderson, 1976; DeKosky and Bass, 1980; Henderson et al., 1980; Terry, 1982). In the final chapter of this book we shall examine the implications of such evidence for the hypothesis of a continuum between aging and dementia.

Glial cells are said to be less affected than neurons (Bolis, 1982), but they may increase in various cortical areas (Brizzee, 1975; Sturrock, 1977). Increase of the gliofibrillary content of astrocytes (fibrous gliosis) is also a characteristic of the aging brain. At the beginning, the increase in fibre content occurs in the molecular layer of the cerebral cortex, but later on may extend to deeper layers. As a result, the microenvironmental homeostasis is supposed to be injured, since glial cells not only have mechanical functions, but play an essential role in the exchange of neurotransmitters and ions in the extra-cellular space. Local dehydration and glial hypertrophy may damage the blood-brain barrier, with further unwanted metabolic consequences (Vernadakis, 1975). Glial cells are less than 40 μm in diameter. The cell bodies of small neurons have a diameter between 40 and 90 μm and large neurons may be greater still.

When Alzheimer's patients and age-matched controls are compared, there are no differences in glial cells and small neurons at mid-frontal, superior frontal and inferior parietal areas. However, in all three areas there are significant decreases in large neurons in the demented patients, with a further lesion consisting of four times as many astrocytes in the layers 2–6 (Terry and Davies, 1983).

Senile plaques are a typical marker of Alzheimer's dementia (Figs. 4.1, 4.2 and 4.3) but they are found even in normal brains (Tomlinson and Henderson, 1976; Terry, 1982). Some histologists have therefore been led to postulate that the conditions are different stages of the same, albeit unknown, process.

Recent observations seem to confirm this view. Generally speaking, the incidence of Alzheimer's dementia is considered to be 5–7% in the population over 65 years, with even lower values (see Chapter 10) in certain countries. Yet

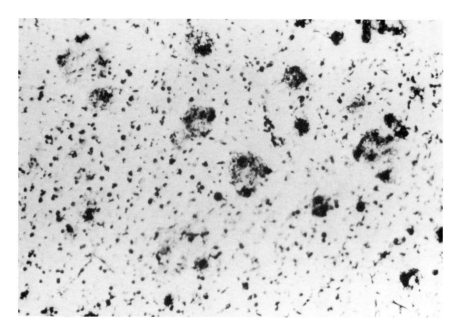

Fig. 4.1   Alzheimer's dementia. Numerous senile plaques, showing a dense core of amyloid and argentophilic halo of fibres and granules. Del Rio Hortega×250. Figs. 4.1–4.5 were kindly supplied by Prof. G. Macchi

Alzheimer-like changes have been reported in brains of 38 out of 51 unselected patients (74.5%) ranging in age from 55 to 64 at the time of death. Within that group 43% had only tangles and 25.5% had both senile plaques and tangles (Ulrich, 1985). Entorhinal cortex and hippocampus were particularly affected. These observations pose intriguing questions. Are these lesions early markers of dementia? Why is there such a difference between clinical epidemiology and autopsy findings? As yet these questions have no answers.

Senile plaques are never found in the cerebellum nor in the spinal cord. Many of them consist of a central core of amyloid with argentophilic cellular debris. They are not quiescent, but have enzymatic activities and contain less tryptophan and tyrosine with a higher carbohydrate content than general amyloid. Thus, the plaques' amyloid is locally formed, probably by microglia, and is not the expression of a general derangement (Powers and Spicer, 1977). There is a negative correlation between plaques and neuronal counts (Mountjoy et al., 1983). It is hard to assess whether cognitive impairment is dependent on the presence of plaques or the declining number of neurons. Perhaps both conditions are necessary.

Plaques form in several stages. At the beginning they are composed of a 'threadlike substance', i.e. few amyloid fibres intermingled with degenerating or dystrophic neurites. The next stage is the classical one with a central core of thick

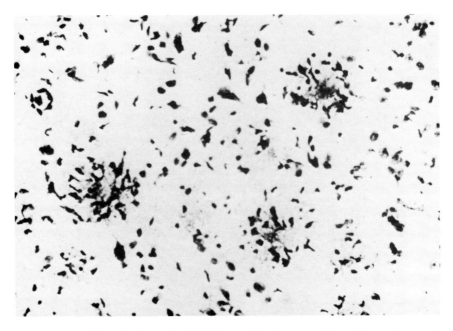

Fig. 4.2 Alzheimer's dementia. Primitive senile plaques with small central core of amyloid and degenerating axons throughout the plaque (×250)

amyloid, surrounded by loosely arranged amyloid fibres and degenerated or regenerating neurites. The final stage is the so-called 'burned-out' plaque, consisting of amyloid which is surrounded by astrocytic elements (Wisniewski et al., 1985).

Microglial cells are always associated with an amyloid deposit. The presence of both the amorphous and fibrillary material at an early stage and its association with microglial cells suggest that the latter are the source of the deposit (Moretz et al., 1983). It is still unclear whether these cells behave as a processor or act as a producer. It is also undetermined whether the chemical composition of the plaques in demented patients is different from that found in apparently 'normal' elderly subjects.

Many attempts have been made to study plaques experimentally in laboratory animals. A typical model of human senile plaques results from the intracranial injection of certain strains of the virus responsible for scrapie in mice (Bruce and Fraser, 1975; Wisniewski et al., 1975 and 1985). These plaques contain amyloid cores, and differ from those induced by intracranial aluminium phosphate. They do not induce inflammatory responses, nor a systemic one. Genetic factors are somehow involved, because only certain strains of mice are susceptible. Probably the endothelial cells of the blood–brain barrier lose their function when they are infected. The possibility of inducing senile plaques has engendered many areas of debate. The question arises as to whether a transmissible agent exists in

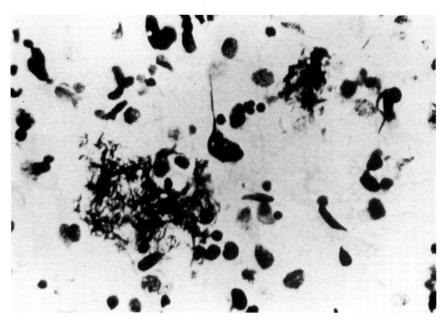

Fig. 4.3   Alzheimer's dementia. A typical plaque with rich argentophilic component. Plaques have a characteristic cycle and are found in apparently 'normal' elderly
subjects. Amyloid is locally formed. There is a negative correlation between plaques
and neuronal counts (×250)

Alzheimer's dementia, as in neurological diseases induced by slow viruses, such as
Creutzfeld-Jakob and kuru. The hypothesis that the plaques are indicative of a
transmissible encephalopathy is currently under investigation (Wisniewski and
Merz, 1985). Certainly the possibility cannot be ruled out that tissue components
of Alzheimer's dementia have a similar toxicity to those of scrapie for either the
amyloidogenetic proteins, associated enzymes or physical compression.

   Senile plaques are not the only expression of amyloid substance in the brain,
because it is found around vessels and in the ependyma. Cerebral amyloidosis is
considered an important expression of changes in the immune system during the
aging process. The localized changes indicate the autonomy of the brain aging
processes. Thus one may find an aging brain without an aging body and vice versa
(Orlovskaya, 1982).

   By means of monoclonal antibodies to choline acetyltransferase (ChAT), a
specific marker of cholinergic neurons, and immunocytochemical techniques,
cholinergic neurites can be identified in the neocortex and in the amygdala of aged
macaques. In some cases, these neurites are associated with the deposit of
amyloid and therefore a link has been proposed between the cholinergic system
and the senile plaques (Kitt et al., 1984). As we shall see in the next chapter, the
finding might be taken to support the cholinergic hypothesis of Alzheimer's
dementia, although this has apparently lost some ground in recent years.

Neurofibrillary degeneration is responsible for the appearance of the tangles (Figs. 4.4 and 4.5). They are typical of Alzheimer's dementia, but are also seen in other types of cerebral pathology, such as dementia pugilistica, von Economo's encephalitis, Guam–Parkinson dementia, subacute sclerosing panencephalitis, and liposomal disorders. Tangles are also found in certain experimental conditions: old monkeys, mice under alcoholic intoxication and neurons in vitro (Crapper McLachlan and DeBoni, 1982). Moreover, almost all old cases of Down's syndrome are affected, supporting the hypothesis of a continuum with Alzheimer's dementia (Mann et al., 1984b). Tangles are lesions within the cytoplasm of the perikaryon of medium and large pyramidal cells of the neo- and paleocortex. They occur less frequently in deep nuclei (Terry, 1980). They are also seen in normal elderly people and raise again the question of a continuum between aging and dementia. Senile plaques and tangles are not present in the same concentrations; plaques may be present without tangles in some individuals. However, both are correlated with the severity of dementia (Terry and Davies, 1983), but it has also been argued that Alzheimer's dementia can occur without histological markers such as plaques and tangles (see McGeer et al., 1984).

The electron microscope makes it possible to identify the structure of the tangle. It is formed of paired helical filaments which differ from normal neurofibres found in the cytoplasm, such as microfilaments, neurotubules and neurofilaments. A normal brain protein in the neurotubule fraction is cross reactive with neurofibrillary tangles and it is smaller than tubulin (Iqbal et al., 1980). How tangles may impair cortical function is unknown. For example, tangles are not responsible for the dendritic loss. A causal relationship between them, as a 'dieback' phenomenon, has not been substantiated (Terry, 1980).

Amyloid, senile plaques and tangles may share a common origin on the basis of an intriguing new hypothesis, that is so far 'but a framework of thought' (Gajdusek, 1985). The neurofilament of 10 nm diameter extends down the whole axon and is composed of three proteins. The structure is not static, but carries enzymes, neurotransmitters and lysosomes to the presynaptic terminal, as a moving fibre. Interference with axonal transport of neurofilaments may cause the appearance of the typical histological markers of Alzheimer's dementia. In fast-conducting fibres, as in spinal neurons, 'ballooning' and death are more likely to occur, whereas in the slower fibres tangles or amyloid are the pre-eminent features. Environmental deficiencies of calcium and magnesium have been the only external identified factor in the world areas having high incidence of motor neurone diseases, parkinsonism with dementia and Alzheimer's disease.

Whatever their action on the cells, senile plaques and tangles are markers of severe brain impairment and both are found in demented people and to a lesser extent in the 'normal' elderly. It is worth noting that demented patients with plaques and tangles appear to have no reduction in the number of synapses, compared with controls (Gibson, 1983), although it must be said that the number of cases in this electron microscopic study was small.

Doubts about age-dependent histological features return when lipofuscin is considered, a pigment that accumulates in the nerve cells and may push the nucleus and the organelles to an eccentric position. The word means black fat.

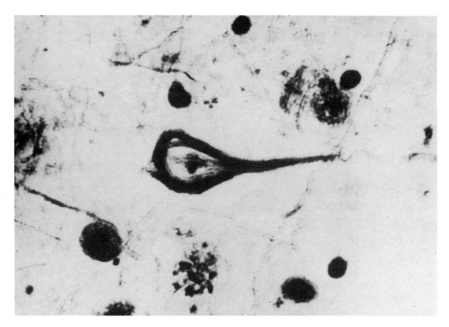

Fig. 4.4   A typical tangle. Tangles are lesions within the cytoplasm of the perikaryon of medium and large pyramidal cells of the neo- and paleocortex, less frequently in deep nuclei (×340)

Histochemical and electron micrographs show the stages of the process (Chang and Pao, 1982). It is found that the oldest cultured neurons have a higher quantity of lipofuscin compared to the youngest ones, thus indicating a correlation with age. Lipofuscin is formed from the cell lysosomes, which are easily identified by their round shape, unit peripheral membrane, homogeneous content and laminated structures. In their biological cycle filaments begin to appear at the region close to the enveloping membrane with a progressive concentric, onion-like lamination. Later on, electron-dense substance occurs only in the laminated part of transforming lysosomes, and in advanced stages the total space of the lysosomes may be filled with thick lipofuscin pigments and few lipid vacuoles. The deposit seems then to diffuse gradually in the cytoplasm, when the outer membrane disintegrates. In the life cycle, the Golgi apparatus may play a major role as a scavenger, thus cleansing the cell, permitting the formation of a new lysosome. When the catabolic process stops in senescence, the residual lipofuscin is no longer removed and accumulates in the cytoplasm. Twenty-eight-month-old human neurons contain no pigment, whereas centenarians may have neurons totally occupied by lipofuscin except for the nuclei (Beregi, 1982). Four types of distribution are identified: 1) no deposit; 2) diffuse distribution; 3) concentration of the pigment at one pole; 4) deposit in the whole cytoplasm pressing the nucleus to one side (Brody and Vijayashankar, 1977). The same authors describe the

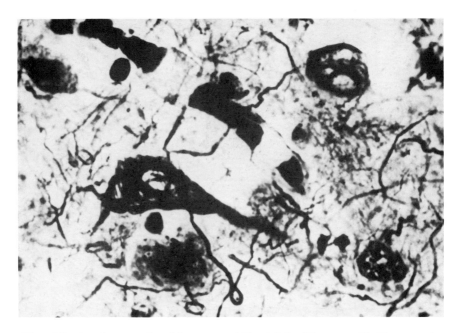

Fig. 4.5 Another tangle with argentophilic debris. The neurofibrillary tangle displaces other organelles. This marker of dementia is due to neurofibrillary degeneration, but is found in other pathological conditions and even in the apparently normal elderly (×340)

presence of numerous amino acids in the lipofuscin. Is the lipofuscin a cytotoxic component or a harmless by-product? It is conceivable that an age-dependent thick deposit inside the cell, pushing the nucleus to an eccentric position, impairs cell function. In adult houseflies the rate of fluorescent age pigment accumulation is significantly faster in short-lived, highly active flies than in long-lived, low-activity flies (Sohal and Donato, 1978). According to these observations lipofuscin would mark the physiological rather than the chronological age. Lipofuscin is found in brain cells of human embryos from schizophrenic women (whether a side-effect of neuroleptics or as a part of the illness is not known), but it is not observed in normal controls (Orlovskaya, 1982).

The proof of lipofuscin cytotoxicity is still lacking. It is argued (Terry and Davies, 1983) that a great deposit of lipofuscin is formed in the inferior olivary nucleus from childhood and yet neurons there are well preserved in the adult (Monagle and Brody, 1974). By contrast, lipofuscin might be beneficial, because it may be part of a system that enables the cell to isolate within a membrane potentially toxic metabolic products and abnormally peroxidized compounds, following a polymerization with lipids and proteins (Terry, 1980). Other studies are also in favour of a strong functional activity, leading to a deposit of harmless by-products (Timiras, 1978). Whatever the role, differences between normal elderly and demented patients are not seen.

It has been suggested that changes in the performance of the so-called blood–brain barrier may have a role in aging. The barrier is believed to exert a control over exchanges between the general circulation and the brain. It consists of 'the endothelial lining cells with their occluding tight junctions, surrounded by a complex basement membrane enfolding scattered perivascular cells, surrounded by a meshwork of astrocyte processes' (Scheibel and Fried, 1983). Few studies have been published so far on its age-variations. Scheibel and Fried report changes observed by means of scanning electron microscopy. The technique provides three-dimensional views comparable to stereological reconstructions of thousands of electron microscopic photographs. In brain from aged animals, and also in the human, a 'dramatic cobblestone' is described, due to pericapillary proliferation, with multiple external protrusions. The aetiology of the massive pericytic overgrowth is unknown. Some of these elements are filled with lipid content and their further fate is obscure. By contrast, in the young individuals the external, abluminal wall is smooth and consists primarily of the basement membrane, with few astrocytes and scattered almond-shaped pericytes. Another stereoscopical study on the capillary net in the human describes an age-dependent increase of some parameters, such as the mean diameter, the capillary volume and the units of cortical volume (Hunziker et al., 1979). Although age-dependent variations of the capillary net and of the pericapillary environment have been described, cerebral blood flow is not dramatically affected in the aged human, as we shall see in Chapter 6. Again, we may find a discrepancy between purely morphological studies and living observations in the elderly. The meaning and effects of so many transformations in the brain tissue with age are far from being understood.

Alterations in the deposit of certain chemical elements have been associated with aging. One of the best known is the aluminium deposit, which is found in the elderly, as well as in Alzheimer's dementia and in dialysis dementia. The injection of aluminium powder into the cerebrospinal fluid of adult rabbits is followed by neurological disorders with prominent spinal involvement (Bugiani and Ghetti, 1983). Early lesions are represented by axon swelling due to accumulation of 10 nm filaments. Neurofibrillary degeneration is seen from the second day on and extends into the dendritic branches. Other experiments in susceptible hosts, such as rabbits and cats, reveal a marked memory and learning impairment in avoidance conditioning a few days after the injection (Crapper McLachlan and De Boni, 1982). Motor disturbances and epileptic status are further complications leading to death. The impairment depends on the neurofibrillary degeneration rather on the aluminium itself, because in rats, mice and monkeys, the neurological signs and the neurofibrillary degeneration are not seen, in spite of a large aluminium deposit. On the other hand, there is a relationship between the severity of the behavioural status and the density of the neurofibrillary degeneration. Research on the generation of action potentials in affected cells indicates a block of the functional transmission from the excitatory postsynaptic potential to the spike, due to a membrane alteration, causing a prolonged depolarization.

The accumulation of other metals has also been studied, including copper, iron and zinc. Doubt exists about their relationship to aging, although zinc is supposed to have a bearing on the aetiology of primary dementia through a disturbance of the availability of glutamate (Constantinidis and Tissot, 1982).

We have so far considered age and disease-dependent pathological changes with little regard for any anatomical localization of the effects. Let us examine the areas and the nuclei that are most affected. One of the sites is the locus ceruleus, a nucleus in the upper pontine reticular formation numbering as many as 19,000 nerve cells (Vijayashankar and Brody, 1979). Its main fibre tracts include an ascending noradenergic bundle and a descending pathway to the spinal cord. Its function is interpreted as a central catecholaminergic system coordinating local changes within the microvessels of the brain and thus minimizing fluctuations in the brain blood flow (Mann, 1983). This author describes the deposit of a pigment, the neuromelanin, within cells of the locus ceruleus from early life increasing linearly with age until about the 60th year. Afterwards, the average pigment level decreases, with the loss of those cells with the highest melanin deposit. The remaining cells are supposed to be more vulnerable to agents of any kind. According to Mann, changes in the now vulnerable central noradrenergic pathways play a role in the pathogenesis of dementia. Most neurons of the pars compacta of the substantia nigra contain a heavy deposit of neuromelanin in their cytoplasm (McNeill et al., 1984). A local degeneration bringing about epinephrin loss is also considered to be related to the parkinsonism associated with dementia (Mizutani et al., 1985). Thus, an age-dependent cell loss occurs in the locus ceruleus, enhanced in cases of Alzheimer's disease by 54% and even more so in cases of parkinsonism and Down's syndrome. The pars cerebellaris seems to be more affected (Wree et al., 1980). On the other hand, no significant difference in the amount of neuromelanin in the locus ceruleus is seen at any age between patients and controls. From this point of view, Alzheimer's dementia and Down's syndrome do not necessarily convey heavier lesions than aging itself (Mann et al., 1984a). By the age of 90 years, the change in Alzheimer's dementia approaches that in old age alone. This statement also stands against the continuum hypothesis. Moreover, the dorsal tegmental nucleus of the raphe complex shows no significant cell loss with age, in contrast to their behaviour in senile dementia (Mann et al., 1984b). Alzheimer's patients dying before the age of 80 years tend to have diffuse cerebral atrophy, with a mean deficit of 12.7%, whereas older patients show rather selective temporal lobe atrophy exceeding that due to age (Hubbard and Anderson, 1981). Also in the group with diffuse atrophy the temporal area is the most affected, being on average 18% smaller than in the controls. Alzheimer's dementia is a disease especially affecting the temporal cortex, which was earlier said to be spared by aging.

Other researches have revealed changes in the basal forebrain, including a rostromedial part sending fibres to the hippocampus and a caudolateral part including the nucleus basalis of Meynert, which sends fibres to the cortex. A sharp decrease in the number of cells in this nucleus is seen in senile dementia (Tagliavini and Pilleri, 1983). In this complex the enzyme choline acetyltransferase (ChAT) is normally present. An age-dependent loss and a parallel decrease in ChAT activity occurs in this cholinergic system; the cell number declines from

450,000 to 140,000 over a normal life span (McGeer et al., 1984). The cholinergic loss is supposed to have widespread and negative effects on cognitive functions and therefore cholinergic therapies have been attempted with various degrees of success.

The data are still debated, because an overall change in cholinergic input to cerebral cortex with age is not confirmed by other authors (Chui et al., 1984). In man neurons in the nucleus basalis of Meynert are easily identified by the large diameter, the prominent single nucleolus and the tendency to form clusters of varying size and shape. A general decline in cholinergic cells in this system should have revealed itself by chromatolysis of these cells in aging brains. This was not observed. The mean density of these cells was 76 neurons/mm^2 uncorrelated with age, thus indicating local stability. Further observations indicate that cell loss in the basal nucleus of Meynert takes place in 75% of cases with Alzheimer's dementia, unrelated to the number of the senile plaques both in the frontal cortex and hippocampal region; the cell loss may therefore play a role, but it is not the primary cause of the disorder (Hirai et al., 1985). On the other hand, neither the quantity of lipofuscin in those cells, nor the quantity of neuromelanin in the locus ceruleus, discriminate patients and controls at any age (Mann et al., 1984a).

Age-related changes in the elderly are found in sympathetic ganglia at cervical, upper thoracic and lumbar levels with increase of lipofuscin, inclusion bodies and lack of tangles (Helèn, 1983). The subjects of this study are not really 'normal', because they are reported to suffer from vascular disturbances; however, the research sheds light on the future opportunity to study biopsy material taken from ganglia for a better diagnosis in undetermined cases. Although spontaneously occurring tangles are rare in animals, they have recently been found in ganglia of aged individuals of the Louvain rat strain. Two main stages have been recognized, the first stage with lipofuscin accumulation and mitochondrial alterations, the second with alterations in the cytoskeleton (van den Bosch de Aguilar and Goemare-Vanneste, 1984).

This chapter has summarized the main anatomical data on the aging brain problem. A picture emerges that justifies the term 'histological drama', one that is parallel to the poetic definition of the 'human ruin that is worse than putrefaction'. Lost neurons, shrinking extra-cellular spaces, transformations in the cytoplasm, bare dendritic trees, a variety of deposits and capillary transformations leave us to wonder how brain tissue retains its own information and masters new knowledge in old age. Yet, technological advances in quantitative histology leave no doubt about the reality of the changes. Moreover, daily experience in CT-scanning shows widening of sulci and ventricles. There is no support at all for the thesis that brain tissue is stable over time.

However we cannot move directly from the anatomical evidence to neuropsychological conclusions. Neuronal loss does not invariably mean cognitive impairment, for two reasons. The first is cell redundancy, the second concerns biological compensation. Cell redundancy means that we use only a small part of our neural inheritance. For example, the undefined span of long-term memory means that man is unaware of his mental capabilities. The loss of cells may account for a reduced capacity to acquire new and unfamiliar information, but does not lead to the loss of previously acquired information, at least not within certain limits. A motivated teenager with a high IQ can learn 10 foreign languages. The same person at the age of sixty years can hardly learn a new one, but can master his own language even better than in adolescence. Thus, even when anatomical changes have occurred, one should not conclude that a mental decline necessarily exists.

The other mechanism involves biological compensation. It means that remaining neurons may take on the functions of those that are lost. In recent years, neural plasticity has attracted much research interest. Axon regeneration, sprouting, presynaptic activation and post-synaptic sensitivity are relatively new concepts that we should carefully consider to provide rehabilitation programmes for the elderly, demented and stroke patients.

Concerning critical sites in the causes of dementia, it seems an oversimplification to point to a single lesion in a small area as the trigger for a disturbance, which lacks a precise psychodynamic course and often differs from subject to subject. For the present, it is worth underlining again that anatomical considerations on their own can be misleading. Let us consider some examples. At the beginning of this century, a famous bandit was found to have a cerebellar malformation. From that observation, theories began as to the effect of brain malformations in producing a 'criminal tendency, with particularly cruel disposition'. Another subject was found by chance to have a cerebellar agenesis. The extraordinary thing is that he worked as a window cleaner in New York yet with this malformation one would have expected a lack of balance.

This chapter began with the caveat that early anatomical studies of aging lack precise data on medical history and neuropsychological assessment. This is difficult enough even today; we shall never have the information to properly classify many of the brains which have been reported as representative of the normal elderly. Perhaps many of the normal specimens displaying tangles and plaques were not psychologically normal at all. On the other hand, it has been argued that Alzheimer's dementia can occur without histological markers such as plaques and tangles. Thus we cannot yet be certain which of the histological changes are age related, which are disease related, whether Alzheimer's is a separate disease, and which features are the primary causes of neuropsychological impairment.

The histological changes we have considered are abnormal in the sense that they are not present in the healthy young adult. If they are abnormal, then aging itself may be regarded as a disease. We shall see in the final chapter that some investigators view aging and dementia as quantitatively different expressions of the same process. What, then, if Alzheimer's disease is due to a slow virus? May aging too be caused by a virus? Beside these paralogisms, which remind us of the ancient sophisms of Greece, it seems right to argue that dementia and natural aging be considered on clinical basis, since the concept of dementia itself is merely psychological and not histological. So far histological and biochemical studies fail to provide a clear differential diagnosis between aging and dementia. Probably, the day is not far off when improved new techniques for analysing spinal fluid for pathological components will make the distinction clear. However, as we shall see, the separation of aging and dementia is already feasible with psychological and electrophysiological methods.

REFERENCES

Balaszi, A. G., Rootman, J., Drance, S. M., Schulzer, M., and Douglas, G. R. (1984). The effect of age on the nerve fiber population of the human optic nerve. *Amer. J. Ophthalm.*, 97, 760–766.

Beregi, E. (1982). The significance of lipofuscin in the aging process especially in the neurons. In R. D. Terry, C. L. Bolis and G. Toffano (Eds), *Aging*, vol. 18. New York: Raven Press, pp. 15–21.

Blinkov, S. M., and Glezer, I. I. (1968). *The Human Brain in Figures and Tables: a Quantitative Handbook.* New York: Plenum Press.

Bolis, C. L. (1982). Neuron-glia interactions and aging. In R. D. Terry, C. L. Bolis and G. Toffano (Eds), *Aging*, vol. 18. New York: Raven Press, pp. 99–113.

Brizzee, K. R. (1975). Gross morphometric analyses and quantitative histology of the aging brain. In J. M. Ordy and K. R. Brizzee (Eds)., *Neurobiology of Aging.* New York: Plenum Press, pp. 401–424.

Brody, H. (1955). Organization of the cerebral cortex. III. A study of aging in the human cerebral cortex. *J. Comp. Neurol.*, 102, 511–556.

Brody, H. (1973). Aging of the vertebrate brain. In M. Rockstein and H. M. Sussman (Eds), *Development and Aging in the Nervous System.* New York: Academic Press, pp. 121–133.

Brody, H., and Vijayashankar, N. (1977). Anatomical changes in the nervous system. In C. E. Finch and S. Hayflick (Eds), *The Handbook of Aging.* New York: Van Nostrand Reinhold, pp. 241–261.

Bruce, M. A., and Fraser, H. (1975). Amyloid plaques in the brains of mice infected with scrapie: morphological variations and staining properties. *Neuropathol. Appl. Neurobiol.*, 1, 189–202.

Bugiani, O., and Ghetti, B. (1983). Effects of prolonged exposure to aluminium on the nervous system. In D. Samuel, S. Algeri, S. Gershon, V. E. Grimm and G. Toffano (Eds), *Aging* vol. 22. New York: Raven Press, pp. 271–275.

Bugiani, O., Salvarani, S., Perdelli, F., Mancardi, G. L., and Leonardi, A. (1978). Nerve cell loss with aging in the putamen. *Eur. Neurol.*, 17, 286–291.

Chang, H. T., and Pao, X. (1982). Lipofuscin pigment formation in cultured neurons. In R. D. Terry, C. L. Bolis and G. Toffano (Eds), *Aging*, vol. 18. New York: Raven Press, pp. 23–31.

Chui, H. C., Bondareff, W., Zarow, C., and Slager, U. (1984). Stability of neuronal number in the human nucleus basalis of Meynert with age. *Neurobiol. Aging*, 5, 83–88.

Constantinidis, J., and Tissot, R. (1982). Degenerative encephalopathies in old age: neurotransmitters and zinc metabolism. In R. D. Terry, C. L. Bolis and G. Toffano (Eds), *Aging*, vol. 18. New York: Raven Press, pp. 53–59.

Corsellis, J. A. N. (1976). Some observations on the Purkinje cell population and on brain volume in human aging. In R. D. Terry and S. Gershon (Eds), *Aging*, vol. 3. New York: Raven Press, pp. 397–398.

Crapper McLachlan, D. R., and De Boni, U. (1982). Models for the study of pathological neural aging. In R. D. Terry, C. L. Bolis and G. Toffano (Eds), *Aging*, vol. 18. New York: Raven Press, pp. 61–71.

Dekaban, A. S., and Sadowski, D. (1978). Changes in brain weights during the span of human life: relation of brain weights to body heights and body weights. *Ann. Neurol.*, 4, 345–356.

DeKosky, S. T., and Bass, N. H. (1980). Effects of aging and senile dementia on the microchemical pathology of human cerebral cortex. In L. Amaducci, A. N. Davison and P. Antuono (Eds), *Aging*, vol. 13. New York: Raven Press, pp. 33–37.

Gajdusek, D. C. (1985). Interference with axonal transport of neurofilaments as a mechanism of pathogenesis underlying Alzheimer's disease and many other degenerations of the CNS. In C. G. Gottfries (Ed.), *Normal Aging, Alzheimer's Disease and Senile Dementia*. Bruxelles: Editions de l'Université, pp. 51–67.

Gibson, P. H. (1983). EM study of the numbers of cortical synapses in the brains of ageing people and people with Alheimer-type dementia. *Acta Neuropathol. (Berlin)*, 62, 127–133.

Gilloteaux, J., and Linz, M. H. (1984). Histology of aging: central nervous system. *Gerontol. Geriat. Educat.*, 4, 81–97.

Haug, H., Barmwater, U., Eggers, R., Fischer, D., Kuhel, S., and Sass, N. L. (1983). Anatomical changes in aging brain: morphometric analysis of the human prosencephalon. In J. Cervos-Navarro and H. I. Sarkander (Eds), *Aging*, vol. 21. New York: Raven Press, pp. 1–12.

Helèn, P. (1983). Fine structural and degenerative features in adult and aged human sympathetic ganglion cells. *Mech. Ageing Dev.*, 23, 161–175.

Henderson, G., Tomlinson, B. E., and Gibson, P. H. (1980). Cell counts in human cerebral cortex in normal adults throughout life using an image analysing computer. *J. Neurol. Sci.*, 46, 113–136.

Hirai, S., Okamoto, K., and Morimatsu, M. (1985). Dementia of the Alzheimer type and the nucleus basalis of Meynert. *J. Neurol.*, 232 (Suppl.), 177.

Hubbard, B. M., and Anderson, J. M. (1981). A quantitative study of cerebral atrophy in old age and senile dementia. *J. Neurol. Sci.*, 50, 135–145.

Hunziker, O., Abdel'al, S., and Schulz, U. (1979). The aging human cortex: a stereological characterization of changes in the capillary net. *J. Gerontol.*, 34, 345–350.

Iontov, A. S. (1984). The morphological basis of age-induced memory changes. *Neurosci. Behav. Physiol.*, 14, 349–353.

Iqbal, K., Johnson, A. B., and Wisniewski, H. M. (1980). Neurofibrous proteins in aging and dementia. In L. Amaducci, A. N. Davison and P. Antuono (Eds), *Aging*, vol. 13. New York: Raven Press, pp. 39–48.

Kitt, C. A., Price, D. L., Struble, R. G., Cork, L. C., Wainer, B. H., Becher, M. W., and Mobley, W. C. (1984). Evidence for cholinergic neurites in senile plaques. *Science*, 226, 1443–1445.

Konigsmark, B. M., and Murphy, E. A. (1970). Neuronal population in the human brain. *Nature*, 228, 1335–1336.

Lintl, P., and Braak, H. (1983). Loss of intracortical myelinated fibers: a distinctive age-related alteration in the human striate area. *Acta Neuropathol. (Berlin)*, 61, 178–182.

Mann, D. M. A. (1983). The locus coeruleus and its possible role in ageing and degenerative disease of the human central nervous system. *Mech. Ageing Dev.*, 23, 73–94.

Mann, D. M. A., Yates, P. O., and Marcyniuk, B. (1984a). Alzheimer's presenile dementia, senile dementia of Alzheimer type and Down's syndrome in middle age form an age related continuum of pathological changes. *Neuropathol. Applied Neurobiol.*, 10, 185–207.

Mann, D. M. A., Yates, P. O., and Marcyniuk, B. (1984b). Relationship between pigment accumulation and age in Alzheimer's disease and Down's syndrome. *Acta Neuropathol. (Berlin)*, 63, 72–77.

McGeer, P. L., McGeer, E. G., Suzuki, J., Dolman, C. E., and Nagai, T. (1984). Aging, Alzheimer disease, and the cholinergic system of the basal forebrain. *Neurology*, 34, 741–745.

McNeill, T. H., Koek, L. L., and Haycock, J. W. (1984). The nigrostriatal system and aging. *Peptides (Fayetteville)*, 5, 263–268.

Meier-Ruge, W., Hunziker, O., Iwangoff, P., Reichlmleter, K., and Sandoz, P. (1978). Alteration of morphological and neurochemical parameters of the brain due to normal aging. In K. Nandy (Ed.), *Senile dementia: Biochemical approach*. New York: Elsevier-North Holland, pp. 33–44.

Mizutani, T., Aki, M., Shiozawa, R., Tanabe, H., Endo, Y., Oda, M., and Hara, M. (1985). Clinico-pathological study of dementia in Parkinson disease. *J. Neurol.*, 232 (suppl.), 25.

Monagle, R. D., and Brody, H. (1974). The effects of age upon the main nucleus of the inferior olive in the human. *J. Comp. Neurol.*, 155, 61–66.

Moretz, R. C., Wisniewski, H. M., and Lossinsky, A. S. (1983). Pathogenesis of neuritic and amyloid plaques in scrapie. In D. Samuel, S. Algeri, S. Gershon, V. E. Grimm and G. Toffano (Eds), *Aging* vol. 22. New York: Raven Press, 61–79.

Mountjoy, C. Q., Roth, M., Evans, N. J. R., and Evans, H. M. (1983). Cortical neuronal counts in normal elderly controls and demented patients. *Neurobiol. Aging*, 4, 1–11.

Murphy jr, G. M. (1985). The human corpus striatum and dentate nucleus: volumetric analysis for hemispheric asymmetries, sex differences and aging changes. *Exp. Neurol.*, 89, 134–145.

Nakamura, S., Akiguchi, I., Kameyama, M., and Mizuno, N. (1985). Age-related changes of pyramidal cell basal dendrites in layers III and V of human motor cortex: a quantitative Golgi study. *Acta Neuropathol. (Berlin)*, 65, 281–284.

Orlovskaya, D. (1982). The process of aging in light of clinical neuropathology. In R. D. Terry, C. L. Bolis and G. Toffano (Eds), *Aging*, vol. 18. New York: Raven Press, pp. 33–41.

Powers, J. M., and Spicer, S. S. (1977). Histochemical similarity of senile plaques of amyloid to apudamyloid. *Virchows Arch. Pathol. Anat.*, 376, 107–115.

Scheibel, A. B., and Fried, I. (1983). Age related changes in the peri-capillary environment of the brain. In D. Samuel, S. Algeri, S. Gershon, V. E. Grimm and G. Toffano (Eds), *Aging* vol. 22. New York: Raven Press, pp. 81–92.

Scheibel, M. E., and Scheibel, A. B. (1975). Structural changes in the aging brain. In H. Brody, D. Harman and J. M. Ordy (Eds), *Aging* vol. 1. New York: Raven Press, pp. 11–37.

Schulz, U., and Hunzinger, O. (1980). Comparative studies of neuronal perikaryon size and shape in the aging cerebral cortex. J. Gerontol., 35, 483–491.

Sohal, R. S., and Donato, H. (1978). Effects of experimentally altered life spans on the accumulations of fluorescent age pigment in the house-fly, musca domestica. *Exp. Gerontol.*, 13, 335–341.

Sturrock, R. R. (1977). Development of the indusium griseum. I. A quantitative light microscopic study of neurons and glia. *J. Anat.*, 122, 521–537.

Tagliavini, F., and Pilleri, G. (1983). Neuronal counts in basal nucleus of Meynert in Alzheimer disease and in simple senile dementia. *Lancet*, i, 469–470.

Terry, R. D. (1980). Structural changes in senile dementia of the Alzheimer type. In L. Amaducci, A. N. Davison and P. Antuono (Eds), *Aging*, vol. 13. New York: Raven Press, pp. 23–32.

Terry, R. D. (1982). Brain disease in aging, especially senile dementia. In R. D. Terry, C. L. Bolis and G. Toffano (Eds), *Aging*, vol. 18. New York: Raven Press, pp. 43–52.

Terry, R. D., and Davies, P. (1983). Some morphological and biochemical aspects of Alzheimer's disease. In D. Samuel, S. Algeri, S. Gershon, V. E. Grimm and G. Toffano (Eds), *Aging* vol. 22. New York: Raven Press, pp. 47–59.

Timiras, P. S. (1978). Biological perspectives on aging. *Am. Sci.*, 66, 605–613.

Tomlinson, B. E., and Henderson, G. (1976). Some quantitative cerebral findings in normal and demented old people. In R. D. Terry and S. Gershon (Eds), *Aging* vol. 3. New York: Raven Press, pp. 183–204.

Tomlinson, B. E., Blessed, G., and Roth, M. I. (1970). Observations in the brains of demented old people. *J. Neurol. Sci.*, 11, 205–242.

Ulrich, J. (1985). Alzheimer changes in nondemented patients younger than sixty-five:

possible early stages of Alzheimer's disease and senile dementia of Alzheimer type. *Ann. Neurol.,* 17, 273–277.

van den Bosch de Aguilar, P., and Goemaere-Vanneste, J. (1984). Paired helical filaments in spinal ganglion neurons of elderly rats. *Virchows Arch. (Cell Pathol.),* 47, 217–222.

Vernadakis, A. (1975). Neuronal-glial interactions during development and aging. *Fed. Proc.,* 34, 89–95.

Vijayashankar, N., and Brody, H. (1979). A quantitative study of the pigmented neurons in the nuclei locus coeruleus and subcoeruleus in man as related to aging. *Int. Neuropathol. Exp. Neurol.,* 38, 490–497.

Wisniewski, H. M., and Merz, G. S. (1985). Neuropathology of the aging brain and dementia of the Alzheimer type. In C. M. Gaitz and T. Samorajski (Eds). *Aging 2000: Our Health Care Destiny.* New York: Springer-Verlag, pp. 231–243.

Wisniewski, H. M., Bruce, M. E., and Fraser, H. (1975). Infectious etiology of neuritic (senile) plaques in mice. *Science,* 190, 1108–1110.

Wisniewski, H. M., Merz, G. S., Wen, G. Y., Iqbal, K., and Grundke-Iqbal, I. (1985). Morphology and biochemistry of Alzheimer's disease. In J. T. Hutton and A. D. Kenny (Eds), *Senile Dementia of Alzheimer Type.* New York: Alan R. Liss, Inc., pp. 263–274.

Wree, A., Braak, H., Schleicher, A., and Zilles, K. (1980). Biomathematical analysis of the neuronal loss in the aging human brain of both sexes demonstrated in pigment preparations of the pars cerebellaris locus coerulei. *Anat. Embryol.,* 106, 105–119.

CHAPTER 5

The neurochemical riddle

There seems to be a reduction in synaptic transmission with age, though the evidence is still confused. Recent research has focused attention on changes in the cholinergic and dopaminergic systems.

Neurochemical investigations of the aging brain are relatively recent, but already the findings are proliferating at a great rate. One finds hundreds of articles in the literature, which consider in great detail individual steps in the complicated and intertwined biochemical processes of the brain. However, most of them deal with animals; few are directly concerned with man. Many of the findings on animals are contradictory and much of the human data is uncorroborated. It is therefore necessary to be cautious in an acceptance of current hypotheses. Problems which complicate the interpretation of the vast literature include the following:

1) the methods used in the various laboratories may be different;
2) the species and the strains of the animals used in the various laboratories also differ, as do the ages at which neurochemical changes have been studied;
3) 'young' and 'old' have different meanings to different researchers;
4) the various groups have studied different brain areas;
5) results obtained from some structures may be biased by the contribution of degenerating, adjacent fibres;

6) old animals are more likely to be ill animals as well;
7) many experiments have failed to control or even specify the gender of the subjects;
8) 'post-mortem' specimens may become degraded in storage or have been influenced by illness or treatment preceding death;
9) variations in receptors and neurotransmitters should be considered in a meaningful context, since the number of receptors is related not only to structural changes, but also to the quality of input.

Let us consider some practical examples of these problems. In a review of cases from three American human specimen banks, a panel of consultants agreed with the hospital record of the diagnosis in only 29% of cases. As a result the panel worked with the National Institute of Mental Health to develop a standard schedule for diagnostic evaluation after death. This is a 180 item inventory, which can be used to establish correlations between clinical data and laboratory findings. This strategy is considered as a necessary stage in improving the reliability of the findings based on post-mortem specimens (Zalcman, 1984). To take another example we have already seen that age has an effect on the number of axons in human optic nerve. The same authors report that the axon count is affected by the delay between death or enucleation and fixation (Balaszi et al., 1984). Likewise, in studies of enkephalin-like immunoreactivity in human hippocampal neurons, post-mortem delay is the major factor affecting the intensity of the localization (Kulmala, 1985). Moreover, the use of animal models presents a particular problem in establishing to what extent the conclusion may extrapolate to humans (Toffano et al., 1984). Among the animal data, there is practically no metabolic marker for any of the neurotransmitter systems where at least two conflicting reports of their variation with age have not been reported (Rogers et al., 1984). It is particularly important to establish at what stage age-related deficits in synaptic transmission occur. Generally speaking, reduction of receptors precedes structural change, but in other cases it is the reverse (Severson, 1984). The change may take place in the availability of the transmitter, or at the receptor or post-receptor levels; few reports are available to localize particular post-receptor alterations responsible for changes in response (Roth and Hess, 1982).

In spite of these difficulties which are characteristic of an emerging field, neurochemical research is becoming a promising scientific discipline. It has probably shown the fastest growth of any area of neuroscience in the last ten years. In this chapter, we shall deal with age-dependent changes in the aging human brain. We shall consider progress and unresolved problems in each area as we go along.

ACETYLCHOLINE

Acetylcholine is considered to play an important role in the maintenance of cognitive functions, even though it is present in small quantities in the central nervous system. Indeed it has been proposed that dementia is primarily a disorder of cholinergic brain mechanisms. The highest concentrations are in the cerebral cortex, in the caudate nucleus, and in parts of the limbic system. The presence of this transmitter is evaluated indirectly by means of either its synthetic enzyme choline acetyltransferase (CAT) or by acetylcholinesterase AChE or by measurement of muscarinic cholinergic receptor density. The molecule is formed by the acetylation of choline and only a minor part is re-utilized following hydrolysis.

A decline in glycolytic turnover decreases the level of acetyl coenzyme A, which is the key substrate for the synthesis of acetylcholine. It has been found that most of the 13 enzymes of the glycolytic pathway are age-independent, but mitochondrial exokinase activity, phosphofructokinase, aldolase and phosphoglycerate mutase decrease in the aging human brain (Meier-Ruge, 1985). A similarity has been pointed out between hypoxia and aging, since cholinergic activity is reduced in both conditions (Gibson and Peterson, 1982). Finally, reduction of respiratory rate impairs the acetylcholine synthesis.

In the human, the data concerning cholinergic changes in the cerebral cortex, hippocampus, caudate and striate are conflicting (Fig. 5.1). Some authors have reported a reduced synthesis of acetylcholine with age, whereas others have failed to confirm such an effect. There are some observations which suggest either an age-related reduction of CAT activity (McGeer and McGeer, 1976; Perry et al., 1977 and 1981) or a lack of variation (Bird and Iversen, 1974; Bowen et al., 1976 and 1983; White et al., 1977; Spokes, 1979; Carlsson et al., 1980; Yates et al., 1980). It is possible that a decrement in CAT activity is higher in demented patients than in age-matched controls. Although the study has no younger controls, the regression line shows that there is a correlation with age in the normal elderly subjects (Sorbi et al., 1980). Higher CAT activity, expressed as μmol/hr/100 mg proteins, is found in the caudate nucleus and in the putamen; lower values are obtained from the hippocampus and the insula. A more recent study reports an age-related decline in CAT activity in frontal cortex in normal elderly people (DeKosky et al., 1985). Other authors argue that both the number of giant neurons in the medial basal forebrain and CAT activity decline with age. CAT levels in the normal elderly decreases from 1.2 μmol/hr/100 mg protein at age 40 to 0.5 at age 95 (McGeer et al., 1984). The authors also argue that dementia symptoms begin when the number of those cells is under 100,000, and that this is responsible for the fall in CAT activity. Some studies support the hypothesis of a selective vulnerability of the cholinergic neurons, which depend on choline originating from the breakdown of membrane phospholipids (Maire and Wurtman, 1984). Owing to conflicting results in neuron counts in the human nucleus of Meynert, as we saw in the last chapter, a possible explanation can be provided by a reduced production of CAT enzyme within these cells.

Attempts have also been made to study age related changes in the cholinergic system by evaluating AChE activity. In this area of research no differences have been reported between demented patients and controls. This technique yields effects which seem to vary independently from CAT activity (Perry, 1980; DeKosky et al., 1985). Age-related variations of AChE activity are unlikely. Explanation appears to be that AChE is not a specific marker of cholinergic activity. Indeed the presence of this substance is not confined to the cholinergic system.

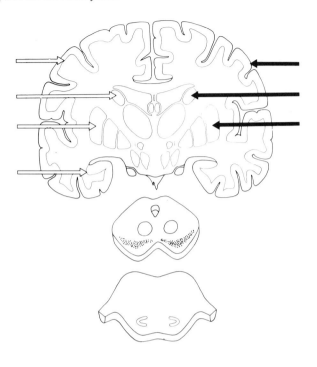

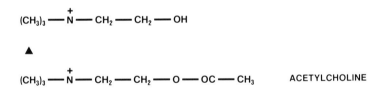

Fig. 5.1 Schematic drawing displaying the contradictory findings in the literature (upper part). The black arrows indicate areas in which acetylcholine decreases with age. The white arrows indicate areas in which this effect has not been found. Synthesis of acetylcholine from choline is also indicated (lower part). The triangle stands for the enzyme choline acetyltransferase

Attempts to confirm the decline in cholinergic activity with age and in dementia on the basis of muscarinic binding have produced conflicting results. A continuous decrease has been reported with increasing age (Enna and Strong, 1981; Nordberg et al., 1982). In the hippocampus the loss of binding sites has an early onset with a sharper decay after the age 50. By contrast, other observations say that muscarinic cholinergic receptor binding is preserved in the whole cortex with age as well as in dementia (Perry, 1980; DeKosky et al., 1985). The distribution of muscarinic binding is the same in all layers of the frontal cortex. Thus, Alzheimer's dementia would be a 'presynaptic' type of mental deterioration. A decrease in the number of nicotine-like binding sites with age is also found (Nordberg et al., 1982).

The decrement in cholinergic activity has been regarded by some authors as the primary factor in the aetiology of Alzheimer's dementia (Drachman and Leavitt, 1974; Drachman, 1977; Bartus, 1979). Stimulation of acetylcholine synthesis and blockade of AChE activity have been considered therapeutic means for improving cognitive functions (Bowen et al., 1983; McGeer et al., 1984), but practical results do not really indicate a successful outcome.

In conclusion, conflicting results have been provided about acetylcholine synthesis, content, inactivation and receptors in the brain. The review of the aging human brain reveals almost as many problems as progress. However, a continuum between aging and dementia is still unproven and the analogy between dopaminergic model in parkinsonism and the cholinergic model involved in memory and cognition may be oversimplistic (Sims et al., 1982). The cholinergic loss is probably a marker of a more generalized pathological process (Kolata, 1983; Coyle et al., 1983; Rossor, 1985). In normal aging, however, metabolism and brain activity stay within the boundaries of a functional reserve, which is certainly lost in dementia.

DOPAMINE

In contrast to the uncertainty about changes in cholinergic system, there is a large measure of agreement on the fate of dopaminergic transmission with age. Moreover there is more direct evidence concerning clinically significant changes in humans. Tyrosine hydroxylase converts tyrosine to dihydroxyphenylalanine (DOPA) and this is the rate-limiting step in the synthesis of catecholamines. DOPA is then decarboxylated to dopamine (DA) by DOPA decarboxylase (Fig. 5.2). Synthesis of dopamine decreases with age in the nigrostriatal system and in the nucleus accumbens (Côte and Kremzner, 1974; McGeer and McGeer, 1976; Adolfsson et al., 1979; Carlsson et al., 1980). A sharp drop is also known to occur in Parkinson's disease (Hornykiewicz, 1974; Riederer and Wuketich, 1976; Lee et al., 1978). Earlier negative findings were due to the use of a control group of 30–40 year olds in whom dopamine levels were already declining (Grote et al., 1974). No age change has been found in tyrosine hydroxylase activity (Robinson et al., 1977). Inactivation by monoamine oxydase (MAO) increases with age (Robinson, 1975; Robinson et al., 1972, and 1977; Grote et al., 1974; Carlsson et al., 1980), especially in the B-form of the enzyme. The increase occurs in MAO-B mostly in nigrostriatal and limbic regions and to a lesser extent in the cortex and medulla oblongata; in contrast, MAO-A activity is steady across the life span (Oreland, 1984). The events are paralleled by changes in binding sites for dopamine which decrease in number in the putamen, substantia nigra and nucleus

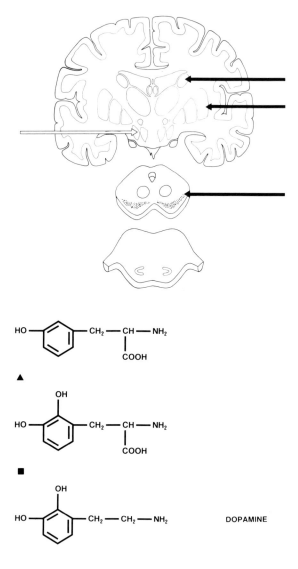

Fig. 5.2 Schematic drawing showing areas where decrease in dopamine with age is found (black arrows). The data are more uniform than those for acetylcholine and there are apparently no changes in the hypothalamus (white arrow). Synthesis of dopamine (lower part) from tyrosine and DOPA is also shown. The triangle stands for the enzyme tyrosine hydroxylase and the square for the enzyme DOPA-decarboxylase

accumbens (Severson and Finch, 1980; Severson et al., 1982; Wagner et al., 1984).

Nowadays, Positron Tomography allows us to identify dopamine receptors in the living human brain, a research approach which is more reliable than studies carried out post-mortem. D2 dopamine receptors (which are not linked or negatively linked to adenylate cyclase) can be imaged in the 43–49 min interval after intravenous injection of labelled 3-*N*-methylspiperone, when binding is facilitated (Wong et al., 1984). Binding to the receptors is estimated by the ratio of radioactivity in the caudate and in the putamen to that in the cerebellum, which contains few or no D2 receptors. A decline in D2 receptor binding with age is found. The authors suggest that there is a decrease in the number of receptors themselves rather than a decline in cerebral blood flow alone. There appear to be sex differences in the decline of receptor binding. For men, the data fit an exponential curve, with a 46% decline in the fitted function over the range 19–73 years. In women, the decline is linear with a 25% decrease in D2 receptor binding over the same period. The quantification of cerebral dopaminergic neurotransmitter function in vivo is in progress at various laboratories, especially in the study of Parkinson's disease (for example Lakke et al., 1985; Leenders et al., 1985; Hågglund et al., 1985; Martin et al., 1985). In patients with Parkinson's disease dopamine concentration is reduced more in the putamen than in the caudate nucleus (Martin et al., 1985), whereas the reverse is true in the normal elderly. In fact, although the caudate nucleus and the putamen have very similar histological and biochemical characteristics, the caudate is more susceptible to aging (Carlsson, 1985).

The decline in D2 receptors in the caudate nucleus with age has been confirmed in 'post-mortem' specimens. By contrast, D1-type binding component (which is linked to adenylate cyclase) increases with age in the caudate (Finch, 1985). A possible explanation is the postdenervation supersensitivity phenomenon consequent upon depletion in the nigrostriatal system.

NOREPINEPHRINE

Dopamine and norepinephrine (NE) have a common origin. NE is synthesized by the action of dopamine-beta-hydroxylase (DBH) on dopamine. As a result, many of the age-dependent changes in DA are also found in NE. DBH activity does not change in the striate nor in the substantia nigra (Grote et al., 1974). The NE content decreases in the brain stem, hypothalamus and hippocampus (Robinson et al., 1972; Robinson, 1975; Carlsson et al., 1980). It does not change in the cortex, striate and thalamus (Carlsson et al., 1980). These data are summarized in Fig. 5.3. Binding sites are decreased in the cerebellum (Corsellis, 1976; Maggi et al., 1979; Enna and Strong, 1981) and locus ceruleus (Vijayashankar and Brody, 1979; Wree et al., 1980), but there is no evidence of a reduction of binding sites in the cerebral cortex. Like dopamine, NE catabolism is accomplished mainly by MAO, and MAO-B increases with age. When the MAO-B activity in Alzheimer's dementia is compared with that of age-matched controls, a significant selective increase is found. The finding would indicate that from this point of view Alzheimer's disease can be regarded as a quantitative exaggeration of normal aging, that is neither uniform nor dependent on a single neurotransmitter (Adolfsson et al., 1979; Carlsson et al., 1980; Oreland, 1984).

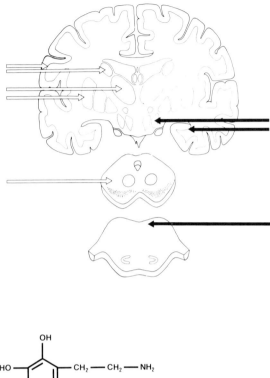

Fig. 5.3 Schematic drawing showing areas where decrease in norepinephrine occurs with age (black arrows). White arrows indicate areas in which the effect has not been found. The triangle stands for the enzyme dopamine-beta-hydroxylase which converts dopamine in norepinephrine

It is thought that binding sites are not stable post-synaptic structures. On the contrary, the lability of such sites is believed to play a central role in the capacity of the nervous system to change its behaviour. Living organisms have adaptive mechanisms and can modulate the number of binding sites for the various neurotransmitter systems. For example, high synaptic activity brings about reduced density of beta-adrenergic receptors. On the other hand, a reduced synaptic input is compensated by a more sensitive post-synaptic membrane. In the aging brain a reduced density of binding sites would reduce the capacity of the system for such adaptive compensation (Freilich and Weiss, 1973). Confirmation of a loss of specific receptors comes from the fact that salbutamol infusions produce only a 50% rise in plasma cAMP in elderly subjects whereas young controls show a 300% increase. The results suggest that the reduced catecholamine responsiveness in elderly subjects is due to a defect in the peripheral beta-receptor-linked adenylate cyclase complex (Ebstein et al., 1984).

SEROTONIN

Serotonin (5-HT) is synthesized in the brain from tryptophan (Fig. 5.4), which is hydroxylated to form 5-hydroxytryptophan and then decarboxylated to form 5-hydroxytryptamine (5-HT). The hydroxylation step is rate-limiting and is apparently quite sensitive to oxygen levels, a point that might be of importance in aging (Rogers et al., 1984). Little is known about age-dependent changes in 5-HT synthesis. The cell bodies in which 5-HT originates are located in the raphe of the brain stem and send both ascending and descending projections. Their content does not seem to change with age in the human brain (Robinson et al., 1972), but 5-HT is high in samples taken from the medulla (Carlsson et al., 1980). Inactivation is probably due to MAO-A (Rogers et al., 1984). Its oxidation produces 5-hydroxyindolacetaldehyde (5-HIAA), a catabolite that significantly increases in cerebrospinal fluid (CSF) with age (Gottfries et al., 1971).

Although there are technical difficulties in the measurement of 5-HT receptor binding, samples of frontal cortex and hippocampus appear to show a reduction of S1 binding sites with age (Shih and Young, 1978; Marcusson et al., 1984a). A decrease in affinity is also reported in the putamen. The S-2a (the authentic serotonergic S-2) binding sites decline with age in the frontal cortex, but not in the hippocampus (Marcusson et al., 1984b). The distribution of serotonin receptors has been imaged and measured by Positron Emission Tomography in the living human brain and the results confirm a decrease with age in both nonspecific and S-2 receptor binding in the caudate nucleus, putamen and frontal cerebral cortex (Wong et al., 1984). Serotonin is known to exert an effect on sadness of mood, anxiety and agitation. The age-related decrease of serotonin over the human life span might account for the frequent depression and sleep reduction in the elderly.

The binding sites for serotonin and indeed for other transmitters may be affected by membrane changes. Changes in turnover and in factors controlling membrane fluidity, for example its phospholipid content, can lead to increased microviscosity and reduce neurotransmitter responses with age (Bonetti et al., 1983).

GAMMA-AMINOBUTYRIC ACID (GABA)

GABA is synthesized from glutamate (Fig. 5.5) in a reaction catalysed by glutamic acid decarboxylase (GAD). Age-changes in GABA are not well known, although it is the most widely distributed neurotransmitter in the central nervous

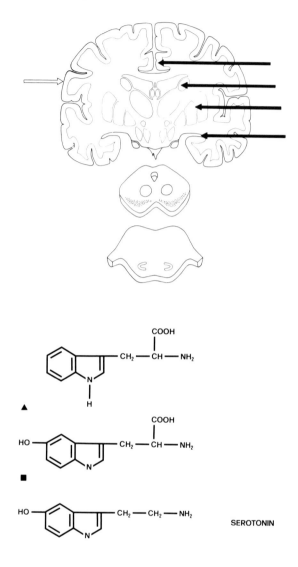

Fig. 5.4 Schematic drawing showing how little is known of age-dependent variations in serotonin in the human brain. The white arrow indicates stability with age.
The black arrow indicates a decrease in receptors. Synthesis of serotonin is also
displayed (lower part), from tryptophan through 5-hydroxytryptophan. The triangle
stands for the enzyme tryptophan-hydroxylase and the square for the successive
decarboxylation

system. The assay of GABA presents particular problems because of its instability
in post-mortem specimens. Accordingly there is some doubt about the reliability
of the available findings. Nevertheless, its synthesis in the human basal ganglia

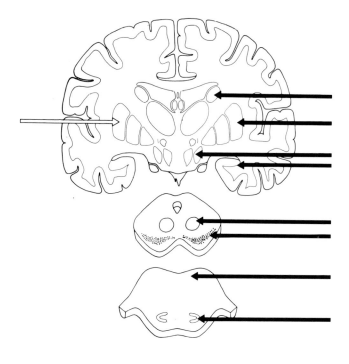

$$HOOC — CH_2 — CH_2 — CH(NH_2) — COOH$$

▲

$$HOOC — CH_2 — CH_2 — CH_2 — NH_2 \qquad \textbf{GABA}$$

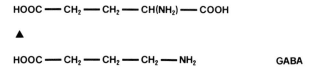

Fig. 5.5   Schematic drawing showing areas where decrease in GABA is seen with age (black arrows). The white arrow indicates areas in which no changes have been found. GABA is synthesized from glutamate (lower part). The triangle stands for the enzyme acid decarboxylase

seems to reduce with age (Côte and Kremzner, 1974; Bowen et al., 1976; McGeer and McGeer, 1976). Similar decrease is also seen in the cerebellum, substantia nigra and hippocampus (McGeer and McGeer, 1976; Spokes, 1979). The putamen is apparently not affected (Bird and Iversen, 1974). It is worth noting that a decrease in GAD is more marked during development than at older ages (Bowen et al., 1976; McGeer and McGeer, 1976). Other regions showing a reduced GABA synthesis are the inferior olive and locus ceruleus (McGeer and McGeer, 1976), amygdala and red nucleus (Spokes, 1979). GABA levels in CSF also decline with age. This age-dependent decline supports the hypothesis of a decreased synthesis of GABA due to the lower GAD activity in some brain areas (Bareggi et al., 1985). These authors found no sex differences in CSF concentration of GABA but Hare et al., (1982) hold that the decrease of this transmitter in lumbar CSF is greater in women. The rostrocaudal concentration is also found to be more pronounced in women, presumably on account of its involvement in neuroendocrine control.

GABA is probably the major inhibitory neurotransmitter in both the brain and the spinal cord. However, too little is known about the function of GABA to be able to relate its age dependent decline to specific changes in neural functions in the elderly.

We shall say little about further neurotransmitters because knowledge of their action in humans is very limited and their changes with age are almost unknown. However, their importance should not be underestimated: it has been suggested that as many as 500 substances can be considered as 'neurotransmitters' or 'neuromodulators'.

Among these substances the neuropeptides have received the most attention. Variations in peptide levels are assessed by their immunoreactivity. Age related changes have been described in somatostatin, but measurements on the temporal lobe indicate that the greatest change occurs before death (Rossor, 1985). Enkephalin-like immunoreactivity is present in the hippocampus without a difference due to aging: it has been mentioned above that post-mortem delay is a major factor affecting its localization (Kulmala, 1985). Beta-endorphin concentrations are apparently similar in elderly and young subjects (Casale et al., 1985). In both groups this study employs the cold pressor test in which a marked increase of plasma beta-endorphin is produced. At 5 min plasma concentration is five times higher than the baseline levels in the young group and 4 times higher in the elderly group. However, the endorphin changes over 10 min is the same in both groups. The results suggest that age does not affect pituitary secretion. In plasma samples beta endorphin shows a typical pattern over the human life span, which follows a paraboloid function, peaking in middle life. By contrast, beta endorphin in CSF shows a linear negative correlation with age (Facchinetti et al., 1983). In the aging rat there are marked reductions in μ and δ receptors, which are independent of one another (Agnati et al., 1984). These changes are of some interest for the endorphins are important in the regulation of pain.

It is worth mentioning a mathematical approach to the fluctuation in certain enzyme levels as a function of age which has been observed in animals. We can fit polynomials to the changes in availability of enzymes described by Benzi et al., (1980), such as malate dehydrogenase and lactate dehydrogenase. There is no linear correlation with age; instead the levels fluctuate displaying a damped oscillation like a sine wave imposed upon a slope (Figs. 5.6 and 5.7). This

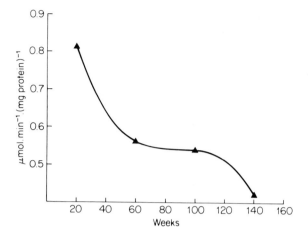

Fig. 5.6   Rat cerebral activity of the enzyme lactate dehydrogenase. Homogenate in toto. The decrease of the enzyme activity is not linear with time, but approximates the polynomial $f(x) = a_0 + a_1x + a_2x^2 + a_3x^2$, thus suggesting regenerative processes. (Adapted from G. Benzi et al., 1980, with permission.)

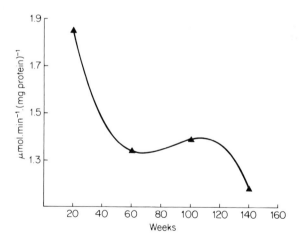

Fig. 5.7   Changes in the activity of the enzyme malate dehydrogenase in the rat cerebrum, homogenized in toto. Same indications as in Fig. 5.6. The curve has the shape of damped waves

observation is important for it suggests that enzymes and perhaps even neurotransmitters may have regenerative cycles, as a consequence of the capacity for compensation which we considered earlier. This opens up the possibility of enhancing such regenerative phases through appropriate pharmacological, dietary and environmental stimulation. In Chapter 12, we shall see how practical advantage can be taken of this principle using neuropsychological methods.

REFERENCES

Adolfsson, R., Gottfries, C. G., Ross, B. E., and Winblad, B. (1979). Postmortem distribution of dopamine and homovanillic acid in human brain, variations related to age and a review of the literature. *J. Neural Transm.*, 45, 81–105.

Agnati, L. F., Fuxe, K., Benfenati, F., Toffano, G., Cimino, M., Battistini, N., Calza, L., and Merlo Pich, E. (1984). III. Studies on aging processes. *Acta Physiol. Scand.*, suppl. 532, 45–61.

Balaszi, A. G., Rootman, J., Drance, S. M., Schulzer, M., and Douglas, G. R. (1984). The effect of age on the nerve fiber population of the human optic nerve. *Amer. J. Ophthalm.*, 97, 760–766.

Bareggi, S. R., Franceschi, M., and Smirne, S. (1985). Neurochemical findings in cerebrospinal fluid in Alzheimer's disease. In C. G. Gottfries (Ed.), *Normal Aging, Alzheimer's Disease and Senile Dementia*. Bruxelles: Editions de l'Université, pp. 203–212.

Bartus, R. T. (1979). Physostigmine and recent memory: effects in young and aged nonhuman primates. *Science*, 206, 1087–1089.

Benzi, G., Arrigoni, E., Dagani, F., Marzatico, F., Curti, D., Polgatti, M., and Villa, R. F. (1980). Drug interference on the age-dependent modification of the cerebral enzymatic activities related to energy transduction. In L. Amaducci, A. N. Davison and P. Antuono (Eds), *Aging*, vol. 3, New York: Raven Press, 113–117.

Bird, E. D., and Iversen, L. L. (1974). Huntington's chorea: postmortem measurements of glutamic acid decarboxylase, choline acetyltransferase and dopamine in basal ganglia. *Brain*, 97, 457–472.

Bonetti, A. C., Battistella, A., Calderini, G., Teolato, S., Crew, F. T., Gaiti, A., Algeri, S., and Toffano, G. (1983). Biochemical alterations in the mechanisms of synaptic transmission in aging brain. In D. Samuel, S. Algeri, S. Gershon, V. E. Grimm and G. Toffano (Eds), *Aging*, vol. 22, New York: Raven Press, pp. 171–181.

Bowen, D. M., Davison, A. N., and Sims, N. R. (1983). The cholinergic system in the aging brain and dementia. In D. Samuel, S. Algeri, S. Gershon, V. E. Grimm and G. Toffano (Eds), *Aging*, vol. 22, New York: Raven Press, pp. 183–190.

Bowen, D. M., Smith, C. B., White, P., and Davidson, A. N. (1976). Neurotransmitter-related indices of hypoxia in senile dementia and other abiotrophies. *Brain*, 99, 459–495.

Carlsson, A. (1985). Brain neurotransmitter in normal aging. In C. M. Gaitz and T. Samorajski (Eds). *Aging 2000: Our Health Care Destiny*. New York: Springer-Verlag, pp. 113–122.

Carlsson, A., Gottfries, C. G., Svenner-Holm, L., Adolfsson, R., Oreland, L., Winblad, B., and Aquilonius, S. M. (1980). Neurotransmitters in human brain analyzed post mortem: changes in normal aging senile dementia and chronic alcoholism. In U. K. Rinne, M. Klinger, G. Stamm (Eds), *Parkinson's Disease*. New York: Elsevier-North Holland, pp. 121–133.

Casale, G., Pecorini, M., Cuzzoni, G., and de Nicola, P. (1985). Beta-endorphin and cold pressor test in the aged. *Gerontology*, 31, 101–105.

Corsellis, J. A. N. (1976). Some observations on the Purkinje cell population and on brain volume in human aging. In R. D. Terry and S. Gershon (Eds), *Aging*, vol. 3, New York: Raven Press, pp. 397–398.

Côte, L. J., and Kremzner, L. T. (1974). Changes in neurotransmitter systems with increasing age in human brain. *Trans. Amer. Soc. Neurochem.*, 5, 83.

Coyle, J. T., Price, D. L., and De Long, M. R. (1983). Alzheimer's disease: a disorder of cortical cholinergic innervation. *Science*, 219, 1184–1190.

DeKosky, S. T., Scheff, S. W., and Markesbery, W. R. (1985). Laminar organization of cholinergic circuits in human frontal cortex in Alzheimer's disease and aging. *Neurology*, 35, 1425–1431.

Drachman, D. A. (1977). Memory and cognitive function in man: does the cholinergic system have a specific role? *Neurology*, 27, 783–790.

Drachman, D. A., and Leavitt, J. L. (1974). Human memory and the cholinergic system. A relationship to aging? *Arch. Neurol.*, 30, 113–131.

Ebstein, R. P., Oppenheim, G., Tropper, S. E., Yagur, A., and Stessman, J. (1984). Hormone stimulated adenylate cyclase activity in aged man and AD/SDAT. *Clin. Neuropharmacol.*, 7 (Suppl. 1), 40–41.

Enna, S. J., and Strong, R. (1981). Age-related alterations in central nervous system neurotransmitter receptor binding. In S. J. Enna, T. Samorajski and B. Beer (Eds), *Aging*, vol. 17, New York: Raven Press, pp. 133–142.

Facchinetti, F., Petraglia, F., Nappi, G., Martignoni, E., Antoni, G., Parrini, D., and Genazzani, A. R. (1983). Different patterns of central and peripheral beta EP, beta LPH and ACTH throughout life. *Peptides (Fayetteville)*, 4, 469–474.

Finch, C. E. (1985). A progress report on neurochemical and neuroendocrine regulation in normal and pathological aging. In C. M. Gaitz and T. Samorajski (Eds). *Aging 2000: Our Health Care Destiny*. New York: Springer-Verlag, pp. 79–90.

Freilich, J. S., and Weiss, B. (1983). Altered adaptive capacity of brain catecholaminergic receptors during aging. In D. Samuel, S. Algeri, S. Gershon, V. E. Grimm and G. Toffano (Eds), *Aging*, vol. 22, New York: Raven Press, pp. 277–300.

Gibson, G. E., and Peterson, C. (1982). Biochemical and behavioral parallels in aging and hypoxia. In E. Giacobini, G. Filogamo, G. Giacobini and A. Vernadakis (Eds), *Aging*, vol. 20, New York: Raven Press, pp. 107–122.

Gottfries, C. S., Gottfries, I., Johansson, B., Olsson, R., Persson, T., Roos, B. E., and Sjostrom, R. (1971). Acid monoamine metabolites in human cerebrospinal fluid and their relation to age and sex. *Neuropharmacol.*, 10, 665–672.

Grote, S. S., Moses, S. G., Robins, E., Hudgens, R. W., and Croninger, A. B. (1974). A study of selected catecholamine metabolizing enzymes: a comparison of depressive suicides and alcoholic suicides with controls. *J. Neurochem.*, 23, 791–802.

Hägglund, J., Aquilonius, S. M., Bergstrøm, K., Eckernas, S. A., Hartvig, P., Langstrøm, B., and Malmborg, P. (1985). Brain 11C-methylspiperone kinetics studied by Positron Emitting Tomography (PET) in patients with Parkinson's disease (PD) and Huntington's chorea (HC). *J. Neurol.* 232 (Suppl.), 9.

Hare, T. A., Wood, J. H., Manyam, B. V., Gerner, R. H., Ballenger, J. C., and Post, R. M. (1982). Central nervous system gamma-aminobutyric acid activity in man. Relationship to age and sex as reflected in CSF. *Arch. Neurol.*, 39, 247–249.

Hornykiewicz, O. (1974). Abnormalities of nigrostriatal dopamine metabolism: neurochemical, morphological and clinical correlations. *J. Pharmacol.* 5 (Suppl.), 64.

Kolata, G. (1983). Clues to Alzheimer's disease emerge. *Science*, 219, 941–942.

Kulmala, H. K. (1985). Immunocytochemical localization of enkephalin-like immunoreactivity in neurons of human hippocampal formation: effects of ageing and Alzheimer's disease. *Neuropathol. Appl. Neurobiol.*, 11, 105–115.

Lakke, J. P. W. F., Vaalburg, W., Paans, A. M. J., Wiegman, T., Kremer, A. M., Rutgers, W., and Korf, J. (1985). Imaging of cerebral DA-receptors in hemiparkinsonism by Positron Emission Tomography. *J. Neurol.* 232 (suppl.), 9.

Lee, T., Seeman, P., Rajput, A., Farlei, I. J., and Hornykiewicz, O. (1978). Receptor basis for dopaminergic supersensitivity in Parkinson's disease. *Nature*, 273, 59–60.

Leenders, K., Palmer, A., Turton, D., Firnau, G., Jones, T., and Marsden, D. (1985). Human cerebral dopamine pathways visualised in vivo. *J. Neurol.* 232 (Suppl.), 9.

Maggi, A., Schmidt, M.J., Shetti, B., and Enna, S.J. (1979). Effect of aging on neurotransmitter receptor binding in rat and human brain. *Life Sci.*, 24, 367–373

Maire, J.C., and Wurtman, R.J. (1984). Choline production from choline-containing phospholipids: a hypothetical role in Alzheimer's disease and aging. *Prog. Neuropsychopharm. Biol. Psychiatry*, 8, 637–642.

Marcusson, J., Finch, C.E., Morgan, D.G., and Winblad, B. (1984a). Ageing and serotonin receptors in human brain. *Clin. Neuropharmacol.* 7 (Suppl. 1), 38–39.

Marcusson, J., Morgan, D.G., Winblad, B., and Finch, C.E. (1984b). Serotonin-2 binding sites in human frontal cortex and hyppocampus. Selective loss of S-2 A sites with age. *Brain Res.*, 311, 51–56.

Martin, W.R.W., Stoessl, J., Adam, M.J., Ammann, W., Bergstrom, M., Harrop, R., Laihinen, A., Rogers, J., Ruth, T.J., Sayre, C.I., Pate, B.D., and Calne, D.B. (1985). DOPA metabolism in aging and in Parkinson's disease: an in vivo study using Positron Emission Tomography. *J. Neurol.*, 232 (Suppl.), 25.

McGeer, E.G., and McGeer, P.L. (1976). Neurotransmitter metabolism and the aging brain. In R.D. Terry and S. Gershon (Eds), *Aging*, vol. 3, New York: Raven Press, pp. 389–403.

McGeer, P.L., and McGeer, E.G., Suzuki, J., Dolman, C.E., and Nagai, T. (1984). Aging, Alzheimer's disease and the cholinergic system of the basal forebrain. *Neurology*, 34, 741–745.

Meier-Ruge, W. (1985). Neurochemistry of the aging brain and senile dementia. In C.M. Gaitz and T. Samorajski (Eds). *Aging 2000: Our Health Care Destiny*. New York: Springer-Verlag, pp. 101–112.

Nordberg, A., Adolfsson, R., Marcusson, J., and Winblad, B. (1982). Cholinergic receptors in the hippocampus in normal aging and dementia of Alzheimer type. In E. Giacobini, G. Filogamo, G. Giacobini and A. Vernadakis (Eds), *Aging*, vol. 20, New York: Raven Press, pp. 231–245.

Oreland, L. (1984). Monoamine oxidase in normal aging and in AD/SDAT. *Clin. Neuropharmacol.*, 7 (Suppl. 1), 32–33.

Perry, E.K. (1980). The cholinergic system in old age and Alzheimer's disease. *Age Ageing*, 9, 1–8.

Perry, E.K., Blessed, G., Tomlinson, B.E., Perry, R.H., Crow, T.J., Cross, A.J., Dockray, G.J., Dimaline, R., and Aggregui, A. (1981). Neurochemical activities in human temporal lobe related to aging and Alzheimer-type changes. *Neurobiol. Aging*, 2, 251–256.

Perry, E.K., Perry, R.H., Blessed, G., Gibson, P.H., and Tomlinson, B.E. (1977). A cholinergic connection between normal ageing and senile dementia in the human hippocampus. *Neurosci. Lett.*, 6, 85–89.

Riederer, P., and Wuketich, S.T. (1976). Time course of nigrostriatal degeneration in Parkinson's disease. *J. Neural. Transm.*, 38, 277–301.

Robinson, D.S. (1975). Changes in MAO and monoamines with human development and aging. *Fed. Proc.*, 34, 103–107.

Robinson, D.S., Nies, A., Davies, J.N., Bunney, W.E., Davies, J.M., Colburn, R.W., Bourne, H.R., Shaw, D.M., and Coppen, A.J. (1972). Aging monoamines and MAO levels. *Lancet*, i: 290–291.

Robinson, D.S., Sourkes, R.L., Nies, A., Harris, L.S., Spector, S., Bartlett, D.L., and Kaye, I.S. (1977). Monoamine metabolism in human brain. *Arch. Gen. Psychiat.*, 34, 89–92.

Rogers, J., Shoemaker, W.J., and Bloom, F.E. (1984). Neurotransmitter alterations in the aging brain. In F.C.A. Visentin (Ed.), *Cerebral Decay*. Milano: Farmitalia–Carlo Erba, pp. 89–124.

Rossor, M.N. (1985). Neuropeptides in human aging and dementia. In C.M. Gaitz and T.

Samorajski (Eds). *Aging* 2000: *Our Health Care Destiny*. New York: Springer-Verlag, pp. 123–130.

Roth, G. S., and Hess, G. D. (1982). Changes in the mechanisms of hormone and neurotransmitter action during aging: current status of the role of receptor and,post-receptor alterations. A review. *Mech. Ageing Dev.*, 20, 175–194.

Severson, J. A. (1984). Neurotransmitter receptors and aging. *J. Am. Geriat. Soc.*, 32, 24–27

Severson, J. A., and Finch, C. E. (1980). Age changes in human basal ganglion dopamine receptors. *Fed. Proc.*, 39, 508.

Severson, J. A., Marcusson, J., Winblad, B., and Finch, C. E. (1982). Age-correlated loss of dopaminergic binding sites in human basal ganglia. *J. Neurochem.*, 39, 1623–1631.

Shih, J. C., and Young, H. (1978). The alteration of serotonin binding sites in aged human brain. *Life Sci.*, 23, 1441–1448.

Sims, N. R., Bowen, D. M., and Davison, D. A. (1982). Acetylcholine synthesis and glucose metabolism in aging and dementia. In E. Giacobini, G. Filogamo, G. Giacobini and A. Vernadakis (Eds), *Aging*, vol. 20, New York: Raven Press, pp. 153–160.

Sorbi, S., Antuono, P., and Amaducci, L. (1980). Choline acetyltransferase and acetylcholinesterase abnormalities in senile dementia: importance of biochemical measurements in human post-mortem brain specimens. *Ital. J. Neurol. Sci.*, 2, 75–83.

Spokes, G. S. (1979). An analysis of factors influencing measurements of dopamine, noradrenaline, glutamate decarboxylase and choline acetylase in human post mortem brain tissue. *Brain*, 102, 333–346.

Toffano, G., Aldinio, C., Aporti, F., Calderini, G., Mazzari, S. and Zanotti, A. (1984). Biochemical models of aging. *Clin. Neuropharmacol.* 7 (Suppl. 1), 14–15.

Vijayashankar, N., and Brody, H. (1979). A quantitative study of the pigmented neurons in the nuclei locus coeruleus and subcoeruleus in man as related to aging. *Int. Neuropathol. Exp. Neurol.*, 38, 490–497.

Wagner, H. N., Wong, D. F., Dannals, R. F., Frost, J. J., Ravert, H. T., Links, J. M., Folstein, M. F., Jensen, B. A., Kuhar, M. J., and Toung, J. K. (1984). Effect of age on dopamine receptors in the human brain. *Clin. Neuropharmacol.* 7 (Suppl. 1), 540–541.

White, P., Hiley, C. R., Goodhardt, M. H.,, Carrasco. L. H., Keet, J. P., Williams, I. E. I., and Bowen, D. M. (1977). Neocortical cholinergic neurons in elderly people. *Lancet*, i, 668–670.

Wong, D. F., Wagner Jr, H. N., Dannals, R. F., Links, J. M., Frost, J. J., Ravert, H. T., Wilson, A. A., Rosenbaum, A. E., Gjedde, A., Douglasse, K. H., Petronis, J. D., Folstein, M. F., et al., (1984). Effects of age on dopamine and serotonin receptors measured by Positron Tomography in the living human brain. *Science*, 226, 1393–1396.

Wree, A., Braak, H., Schleicher, A., and Zilles, K. (1980). Biomathematical analysis of the neuronal loss in the aging human brain of both sexes demonstrated in pigment preparations of the pars cerebellaris locus coerulei. *Anat. Embryol.*, 106, 105–119.

Yates, C. M., Simpson, J., Maloney, A. F. J., Gordon, A., and Reid, A. H. (1980). Alzheimer-like cholinergic deficiency in Down syndrome. *Lancet*, ii, 979.

Zalcman, S. (1984). Diagnostic issues in the use of postmortem material in neuropsychiatric research. *Clin. Neuropharmacol.* 7 (Suppl. 1), 921.

CHAPTER 6

CT scan, CBF, PET and NMR

New technologies promise to clarify the issues.

CT SCAN

Computed Tomographic scan (CT scan) has proved its value many times in gerontology by establishing a proper diagnosis that eluded traditional methods. For instance it has often shown that an apparently senile dementia is secondary to a brain tumour or to a normal pressure hydrocephalus. CT scan has therefore been welcomed by neurologists, psychiatrists and neurosurgeons, as a useful instrument for the study of brain morphology in the elderly patient, in reference to pneumoencephalography, for example, which is invasive, painful and difficult to interpret. Yet after several years experience with the technique, we have to conclude that its contribution to clarifying aging problems has not been very great. Indeed, careless examination and lack of normative data have sometimes led to incorrect radiological evaluations. Much grief has been caused by the use of the word 'atrophy' in descriptions of the brains of neurotics and normal subjects. Part of the problem is that radiologists may tend to go beyond the limits of description, to infer irreversible pathological processes, sometimes spuriously.

CT scan has shown age-dependent widening of sulci and ventricular dilatation. (Fig. 6.1). Changes occur early in human life. Around the 40s the third ventricle

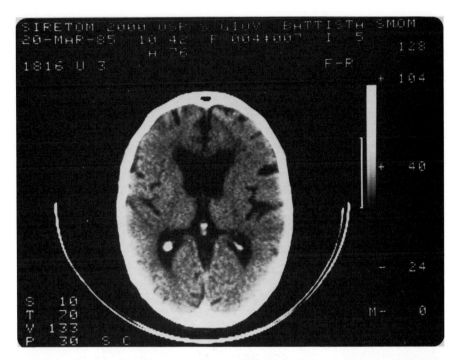

Fig. 6.1 Section of a CT scan passing through the lateral and third ventricles in a subject aged 76, apparently normal. Dilatation of sulci and ventricles. No cognitive impairment. (Figs. 6.1–6.4 were kindly supplied by Drs. G. L. Paroni Sterbini and F. M. Solivetti)

begins to appear larger, from 2 to 4 mm, but the anterior end of the sylvian fissure and the anterior end of the interhemispheric fissure can be as large as 2 mm even in the 30s, when superficial sulci can be 3 mm wide or more (LeMay, 1984). There are, however, marked interindividual differences, some of which are inversely correlated with life span. The brain atrophy index (BAI) and CSF space volume increase exponentially with age, from the 30s on (Takeda and Matsuzawa, 1984). BAI (%) is expressed as 100% × (cerebrospinal fluid space volume/cranial cavity volume). A sex-difference is also found. While in men there is a 1% increase in BAI in the 40s, women of the same age show an 0.5% increase, but, from the 40s on, BAI increases more and more although the mean value is higher in men at least until age 80. The brain stem too appears reduced in size (Steiner et al., 1985).

The BAI can double in 19.4 years in men and in 17.4 years in women. While the rates of increase of both CSF space volume and BAI accelerate constantly over the female life span, the rate in men is particularly high in the 30s and 40s, more than twice that of women of the same age. Later on it declines and accelerates constantly after the 50s until the 80s, as in women.

Thus, after the third decade the loss of brain tissue progresses as if it followed the course described by the Gompertz equation. Brain cells die, as the human population does, in geometrical progression with a constant ratio within equal successive intervals: a straight line of logarithmic scale.

Another measure used by some scanners is the Free Space Volume Index. The value is expressed as 100% × (free space volume/cranial cavity volume). It begins to increase only in the 60s (Zatz et al., 1982; Takeda and Matsuzawa, 1985).

Other studies stress the importance of combined parameters as markers of brain loss. They are linear, such as the bicaudate ratio, sylvian fissure ratio, the third ventricular brain ratio and prepontine–pontine ratio. The simple and the weighted summation of some ratios is considered a suitable method for assessing changes in brain volume (Gomori et al., 1984).

In normal aging the widening of the sulci is greater than that of the ventricles, but in Alzheimer's dementia (Figs. 6.2 and 6.3) the opposite seems to occur

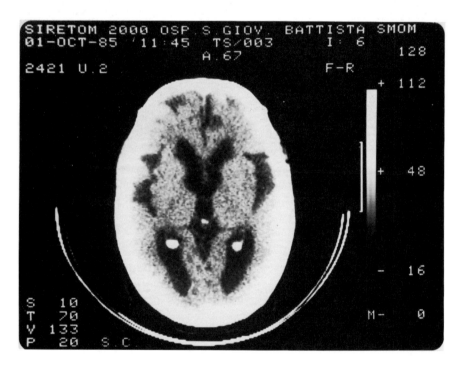

Fig. 6.2   CT scan in a 67-year-old patient suffering from Alzheimer's dementia. The sulci and ventricles are clearly enlarged, but visual examination does not permit judgements of the mental level, since it is dubious whether CT scan can be used to discriminate demented from normal elderly subjects

(DeLeon and George, 1983). All these increases in fluid spaces are correlated with age, but generally not with mental decay (Earnest et al., 1979; Kaszniack et al., 1979; Angeleri et al., 1983). It is therefore hazardous to make the diagnosis of dementia in a patient without reference to the clinical state. This has so far proved to be the case (Masdeau and Aronson, 1985), although some partial

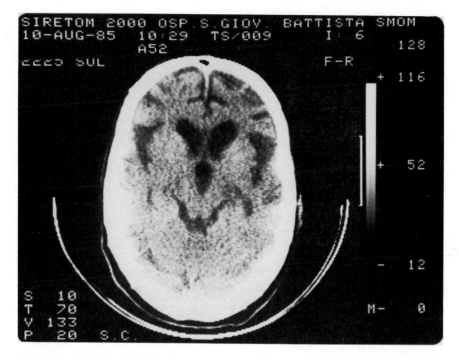

Fig. 6.3 CT scan in a 52-year-old patient suffering from Alzheimer's disease. Severe dilatation of the lateral and third ventricle

correlations between CT scan and the Luria-Nebraska test of mental functions have been found (McInnes et al., 1985).

In centenarians, the mean ventricular brain ratio was found to be 9.4% greater than in a control group having a mean age of 67 years (Goldstein et al., 1985). The variation was considerable and three out of 10 subjects in this age group had mild periventricular white matter lucency. Yet, mental status tests failed to demonstrate mental decline in any of them. Seven of the 10 centenarians had very well-preserved mental capabilities: thus, the relationship between brain atrophy and cognitive function is still unclear. Other reports deny the possibility of discriminating aging and dementia (Yamamura et al., 1980; Brinkman et al., 1981). The authors use as significant parameters bifrontal and bicaudate lines, the widening of the four major sulci, a ventricular area of cella media, the third ventricle and the sylvian fissure.

Among all these structures, the third ventricle and the surrounding structures are those potentially most significant (De Leon and George, 1983). However, these authors question the CT scan approach to aging because: 1) there is a lack of normative data, 2) subjects with negative CT scan and subjective complaints are considered as 'normal', 3) there are too many linear measures where volume would be more appropriate, 4) there is poor comparability, 5) there are no generally agreed standards on equipment and methodology, 6) skull and parenchyma can obscure sulci by what is known as 'partial averaging', 7) sulci are irregular and difficult to measure.

Other recent studies are more optimistic about the possibilities of separating elderly and demented subjects. On the slice at the maximum width of the lateral ventricles, a measure of the mean CT density of parenchyma correctly predicts the group membership in 77.42% of subjects. A second parameter, the fluid volume improves discrimination to 93.55% (Albert et al., 1984a and b).

In the study of aging and dementia, the validity of CT scan data is also challenged by the speed of venticular dilatation and widening of the sulci. Correlations between mental capabilities and atrophic areas are probably dependent on the rate of the change in the tissue and on the site of the affected area. At present, there is no standard methodology for assessing this rate of change. In some cases localized atrophies do explain some of the neurological signs. For example, the CT scan of Fig. 6.4 refers to a patient with a severe impairment of

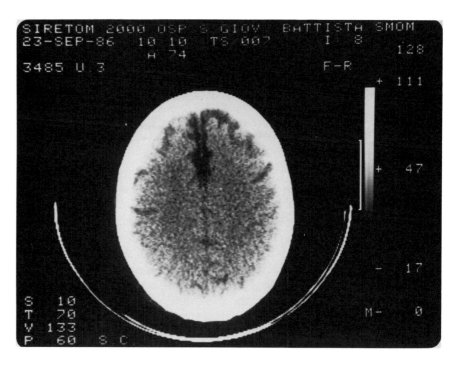

Fig. 6.4 Wide interhemispheric fissure at frontal level in a 74-year-old patient with extrapyramidal signs and complete apathy. Ventricular dilatation was not particularly marked

psychomotor activities and loss of autonomous behaviour. The global atrophy was not very severe, except for that at the level of the interhemispheric surface of the frontal lobes.

In conclusion, CT scan shows age-dependent changes and there are sex differences in the rate of those changes. However, the relationship between morphological data and cognitive impairment is still uncertain. At present, it is therefore unwise to make a diagnosis of dementia on the basis of CT scan alone.

CEREBRAL BLOOD FLOW

The study of cerebral blood flow (CBF) began with confident claims several decades ago. Although it is by no means an obsolete technology, its contribution to the interpretation of aging and dementia processes has been poor and we shall see that it has so far failed to reach any definite agreement.

Basically there are two cohorts of thought. One, originating in the early 1980s, takes the view that CBF declines with age. The other, swayed by more recent findings, is less certain that such an effect occurs except as a secondary effect of disease processes. Many authors argue that CBF reduces with age. The flow, albeit reduced, is coupled to a similar reduction in cerebral metabolic rate for O_2, $CMRO_2$ (Frackowiak et al., 1984a; Lenzi and Pantano, 1984). The reductions in CBF and $CMRO_2$ are not great, being respectively -17% and -10%, whereas the oxygen extraction rate (OER) is increased. A study on volunteers has shown a negative correlation between CBF and age, at the rate of about 4.9 ml/100 ml per minute per decade, but $CMRO_2$ lacks any clear correlation with age (Frackowiak et al., 1984a). OER is also not really age-dependent, in spite of the forementioned increase in the elderly group compared to that of younger controls. If the data on the OER increase are reliable, that is to say, if they are not influenced by cerebral blood volume (CBV), then an important compensating mechanism for a falling CBF has been identified. An increased OER is considered as a risk factor (Fieschi and Lenzi, 1983), because it may mean that the brain tissue has a reduced capacity to be aided by reserve strategies, when ischaemic attacks occur. Except under such critical conditions, however, oxygen reserve has a satisfactory response to metabolic demand even in the elderly. Preserved regulation of oxygen supply to metabolic demand supports earliest observations in the elderly (Lenzi et al., 1981). A modest increase in OER does not imply a state of chronic ischaemia, since there is over 50% of unextracted venous oxygen available to the brain (Frackowiak et al., 1984b).

The reduction in CBF in the elderly and perhaps also $CMRO_2$ to a lesser extent was supported by other observations. Decreases of local CBF are the highest in frontal cortex, followed by basal ganglia, prefrontal cortical area and by motor and premotor areas (Tachibana et al., 1984a). The white matter is less affected as are the anterior speech and visual areas, sites of long-lasting abilities in the human life span. In patients suffering from either multi-infarct dementia (MID) or Alzheimer's disease (AD) mean grey matter flow is reduced compared to that in age-matched normal controls. Unlike MID, AD shows no age-dependent decrease in flow values, but reduction of CBF is significantly correlated with the severity of dementia (Tachibana et al., 1984b). Hyperfrontality, a higher CBF in frontal areas at rest, also has a tendency to decrease with age. According to other researchers (Pantano et al., 1984a), it occurs mainly in the grey matter.

The finding is probably due to neuronal loss, or alternatively, to functional changes, such as programming motor activities and conditioning emotions. White matter CBF and $CMRO_2$ values are quite stable with age perhaps because glial cells are less affected than neurons. In these frontal regions, the hemispheres appear to be affected equally (Tachibana et al., 1984a; Pantano et al., 1984a). In temporal regions, on the other hand, a reduction of CBF has been identified in the left hemisphere of normal subjects, which is not associated with risk factors for vascular disorders (Zemcov, et al., 1984; Dupui et al., 1984). This may correspond with some EEG phenomena, which are confined to the left hemisphere in a normal population.

Progressive CBF decline has been confirmed both by the usual cross-sectional methodology and by longitudinal studies over a four-year period (Shaw et al., 1984). From the 40s on, CBF declines at the rate of 0.5 ml/100 g/min per year. The reduction does not affect all regions equally. The most affected area is, again, the prefrontal one, followed by parietal, inferior temporal, motor and fronto-temporal areas. Some regions, for example, the occipital lobe, are not affected by aging. Another longitudinal study examined the modification of cerebrovascular reactivity over a four-year interval, by comparing changes in grey matter CBF during steady state breathing of room air followed by 100% oxygen inhalation. It was found that cerebral vasoconstriction reduces linearly from middle age to old age in normal subjects (Rogers et al., 1985). The authors suggest that the decline is due to the increasing rigidity of brain vessels secondary to arteriosclerosis, but other mechanisms are also involved such as decrease of O_2 consumption, CO_2 production and changes in the abundance of neurotransmitters.

A steep decrease in CBF can be seen even in subjects in their 30s indicating that the phenomenon is not confined to old age (Globus et al., 1984). In the next decade, CBF is reduced by a further 11% and we have seen that CT scan observations similarly reveal clear changes at age 30, with a further increase at age 40, especially in men. From other data one can see a reduction of cortical blood flow even in a cohort having a mean age of 24, compared to one with a mean age of 13 years (Dupui et al., 1984). Obviously, the difference is more pronounced when comparison is made between the young and the old subjects. After the age of 60, it is held that autoregulation is no longer maintained, probably because of a rise in cerebral prostaglandins or a defect in parasympathetic activity (Oiwa et al., 1984). A multiple correlation analysis shows that age is the most important factor determining CBF decline with a 0.34 correlation coefficient, followed by lower values for blood sugar, haematocrit, cholesterol, systolic blood pressure, fibrinogen, uric acid, platelets and so on (Shinohara et al., 1984).

Lassen and Ingvar (1980) play down the role of ischaemia in the aging brain and rule out a hypothetical preventive role of vasoactive drugs. Environmental stimuli do have an influence on CBF (Kobayashi et al., 1984). When individual psychophysical characteristics are considered, other than the usual risk factors, a delay in the decrease of CBF with age is observed in active subjects. On the other hand, lack of stimulation can have effects even in younger individuals living in poor conditions. The authors argue that social stimuli can slow down the aging process, confirming other observations. Monetary reward enhances CBF in normal elderly subjects performing arithmetical tasks, precisely in those areas which show lowered perfusion compared to young controls (Warren et al., 1985). Average CBF can apparently be lower in the normal elderly than in control subjects and a decline in flow in demented patients is more severe than the clinical state would suggest. In patients with progressive dementia the rate of CBF decrease can be from 5 to 150 fold greater than that expected in normal aging with a tendency for a more rapid decline in MID patients (Barclay et al., 1984). Finally, in Parkinson's disease a steep decrease in CBF is seen which is largely independent of age, but which correlates with the dopaminergic loss and therefore with the severity of the disease (Tachibana et al., 1985).

Unfortunately, studies of CBF and cerebral metabolism do not all point in the directions so far outlined and there is no general agreement on the main issues. Technical bias, differences between the effects in grey and white matter, different populations and silent pathology can obscure CBF decline, leading to conflicting observations from different research groups. For example, Dastur (1985) has found no evidence for changes in CBF or $CMRO_2$ over the human life span, provided subjects are healthy and active in their environments. In two cohorts with mean ages of 71 and 21, no significant difference is found in CBF and $CMRO_2$. Strangely, one finds from these data that CMR_{glc} is maintained in normal subjects with hypertension as it is in normotensive arteriosclerotic subjects, who show a CBF decline. On the contrary, there is a significant decline of 23% in CMR_{glc} in the elderly group, as we have already noted (Gottstein et al., 1970). That research indicates a possible utilization of ketone bodies as an alternative substrate for oxidative metabolism.

Hyperfrontality is still observed at advanced age, provided that subjects are free of circulatory problems (Mamo et al., 1983). It is worth noting that the authors see a better stability in women, a finding that will become important, when we look at the electrophysiological data. The stability of CBF in the grey matter of females at least until they reach their 50s, has been attributed to an anti-aldosterone effect of their elevated progesterone levels (Meyer and Shaw, 1984). Thereafter, values for women decrease more rapidly and approach those of men. The aforementioned sex-dependent variations seen by CT scan (Takeda and Matsuzawa, 1984) show more or less the same trend.

The normal elderly have also been found to have the same CBF as young controls in a study that used computerized EEG analysis as a basis for assessing healthy cortical function (Dekoninck et al., 1982). Other studies report little or no age-related reductions in vasomotor reactivity associated with normal aging (Davis et al., 1983). Similarly Hartmann and Reis (1985) found no variations of mean CBF with age, when patients with vascular damage, or at risk of it, were excluded.

In summary, the early conclusion that both CBF and cerebral metabolism decline with age has to be revised in the light of recent evidence (Table 6.1). Uncertainty over age changes in CBF has led to opposite lines of 'cerebral philosophy' (Fieschi and Lenzi, 1983). The first, a nihilistic one denies any validity to CBF studies, while the second approach is technological and calls for new models and better equipment.

Table 6.1 Synopsis of some contradictory findings in the literature

CBF

Decrease	Dupui et al., 1984; Frackowiak et al., 1984; Globus et al., 1984; Lebrun-Grandie et al., 1983; Pantano et al., 1984; Shaw et al., 1984; Shinohara et al., 1984; Tachibana et al., 1984; Warren et al., 1985; Zemcov et al., 1984.
No change	Lassen and Ingvar, 1980; Dekoninck et al., 1982; Dastur, 1985.

CMRO$_2$

Decrease	Gottstein et al., 1970; Kuhl et al., 1984; Pantano et al., 1984.
No change	Dastur, 1985; Duara et al., 1983.

CMR$_{glc}$

Decrease	Kuhl et al., 1984; Dastur, 1985; Riege et al., 1985.
No change	Cutler, 1985; De Leon et al., 1985; Duara et al., 1983; Ferris et al., 1983; Rapoport et al., 1984.

POSITRON EMISSION TOMOGRAPHY

Positron Emission Tomography (PET) is currently employed to examine local cerebral metabolism and blood flow in the cortex as well as in deep structures. This new technique images regional brain function, not structure (Fig. 6.5).

Rates of regional glucose utilization in young and elderly normals do not display significant differences at the level of the basal ganglia (Ferris et al., 1983). On the other hand, glucose utilization is significantly reduced in these structures in patients with Alzheimer's disease compared with age-matched elderly controls in normal health. By averaging the rates in sections passing through the caudate nucleus and the thalamus (including other structures at that level such as the white matter and temporal areas) there is a 20.53% decrease in the Alzheimer's group. At the level of centrum semiovale, a 26.43% mean decrease is seen, by averaging frontal, parietal and white matter regions on both sides. Finally, the authors find significant correlations between the rates of glucose utilization and cognitive impairment in memory tasks and in some items of the Wechsler Adult Intelligence Scale (WAIS).

Other PET studies have shown that mean CMR$_{glc}$ decreases gradually with age. On average, at age 78 the rate is 26% less than that at 18. The slopes of decline are similar over areas corresponding to centrum semiovale, caudate, thalamus and overall frontal, temporal, parietal and occipital cortex. White matter CMR$_{glc}$ shows a similar significant decline with age (Kuhl et al., 1984). The authors argue that ventricular dilatation does not cause an underestimation of mean CMR$_{glc}$ nor does it explain the magnitude of the decline, since corrections are made for these factors. Age changes in the rate constants for membrane transport and phosphorylation processes have no major effects on the measurement of local CMR$_{glc}$. Research on the correlation among measures of memory and regional brain glucose metabolism indicates an age-dependent decline in Broca's area (Riege et al., 1985). Low but detectable correlation was found

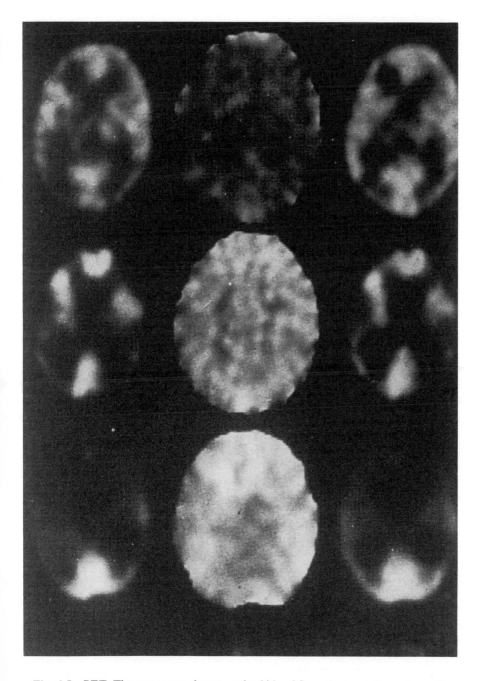

Fig. 6.5 PET. The upper row shows cerebral blood flow, the second row shows O_2 extraction and the third one the O_2 utilization. The first column, refers to a patient suffering from multi-infarct dementia, the central column to a normal volunteer and the third to a patient suffering from Alzheimer's dementia. Right hemispheres are on the right side. The illustration has been kindly supplied by Prof G. L Lenzi

between certain brain areas and test scores. High scores in the WAIS block design test, reconstruction of sentences and immediate memory for a story are associated with high metabolism in the superior frontal areas.

Unfortunately, this field encounters a number of methodological problems which have not yet been settled. The early conclusions concerning brain metabolism in the aged have been questioned on the grounds of incomplete experimental design (Rapoport et al., 1984). They hold that no aging study has examined healthy subjects in the resting state, without visual and auditory input. Sensory input activates not only primary projection areas, but also the rest of the brain. Since hearing and vision are reduced with age, the different cohorts are not equated and so values from the elderly group may be underestimated. CBF does not decline with age if basal levels are measured when the subject's eyes are covered and ears plugged with cotton. Rapoport et al. (1984) show that age differences are not found for regional CMR_{glc} even in normal elderly if measurements are made under these conditions. Finally, there is no correlation between measures of cognitive function and the resting CMR_{glc}.

The lack of any significant relation between CMR_{glc} and age has been supported by Duara et al. (1983) and Cutler et al. (1984). They examined normal subjects between the ages of 21 and 83, who were carefully screened to exclude those with neurological, psychiatric and physical disorders. The subjects were examined with eyes closed and ears plugged. This contrasts with other studies of normal subjects of a similar age range, evaluated with PET scanning but with ears unplugged, in which a decrease in CBF and $CMRO_2$ has been found (Lebrun-Grandie et al., 1983; Pantano et al., 1984b). A great deal of attention must now be paid to variables such as the health of the subjects, sensory influences and psychological conditions in the design and interpretation of PET studies.

The age invariance of basal brain metabolism does not fit with the morphological and biochemical changes that have been discussed in previous chapters. For example, PET studies fail to show any decline of glucose utilization in several cortical areas in spite of the widening of the sulci. Compensatory mechanisms of neuronal plasticity such as increased dendritic growth may account for this paradoxical finding (Cutler, 1985). These mechanisms must be responsible for the maintenance of cognitive functions in the elderly in spite of morphological involution.

Normal subjects with a mean age of 67 have a 14% increase in ventricular size that is uncorrelated to any change of glucose metabolism in the surrounding tissue (De Leon et al., 1985). By contrast, in AD patients there is an 11% increase in ventricular size related to age-matched controls which is associated with a 23% decline in local glucose metabolism. The discrepancies between PET findings and brain atrophy in the normal elderly may be accounted for by the fact that regional CMR_{glc} and $CMRO_2$ are rates per 100 g tissue but not rates for the whole brain (Rapoport et al., 1984). Thus, global measurements which include metabolically inactive fluid spaces may influence the volume over which the PET measurement is averaged and the error may vary among subjects. A technique to correct for potential errors is described (Herscovitch et al., 1984).

In conclusion, the major result from recent PET studies is the lack of change in cerebral metabolism with aging, at least in baseline measurements with low sensory input. Chronic ischaemia can therefore no longer be considered a mechanism responsible for the aging of the brain.

Although a controversial issue, PET studies seem to indicate that the decline in CBF and $CMRO_2$ is gradual, small and generalized, without evidence for a selective, focal 'aging pathology' (Frackowiak et al., 1984a). However, sensory input certainly affects the results. Findings of clinical differences and receptor identification, as described in the previous chapter, permit us to foresee further advances in the near future with better knowledge of neurochemistry and neuropharmacology.

NUCLEAR MAGNETIC RESONANCE (NMR) (see Fig. 6.6)

As yet there are insufficient observations of the aging brain to assess the value of NMR in the study of the aging processes. NMR eliminates the use of ionizing radiation and provides tomograms of the head in any view. The NMR for hydrogen detects the water content of tissue. Pathological features of the white and grey matter are more clearly visualized in NMR images than in CT scans. A third of AD patients display abnormalities of the periventricular white matter. The meaning of this is still unclear (Bryan, 1985) though they may represent vascular pathology (De Leon et al., 1985). This hypothesis is supported by the finding of alteration in the white matter in 100% of patients clinically diagnosed as having dementia of vascular origin (Erkinjuntti et al., 1985). An important contribution of NMR is an improvement in the differential diagnosis of MID and AD. However, for the reasons we considered when discussing CT scan, it is unlikely that observations on gross brain morphology will greatly enhance the understanding of the aging process itself, even with the improved resolution of NMR.

In the early chapters of this book we saw that aging was a process accompanied by loss of neurons, widening sulci, dilating ventricles and the accumulation of useless tangles and plaques within the brain's neural network. At the cellular level there were membrane changes, genetic errors and a reduction in the availability of transmitter substances in the organization of mental activity. It began to look as if aging was indeed 'a ruin worse than putrefaction'. Now we see that in spite of these structural changes, baseline CBF, $CMRO_2$ and CMR_{glc} and their response to stimulation hold up to a large extent so long as other, identifiable disease processes are not at work. These factors will prove important in extending the competence of this growing segment of society. Clearly, the new imaging technologies have told us more that is hopeful about the preservation of function than they have about the declining architecture of the brain, but both approaches are necessary for an understanding of all the changes (Benton and Sivan, 1984).

82

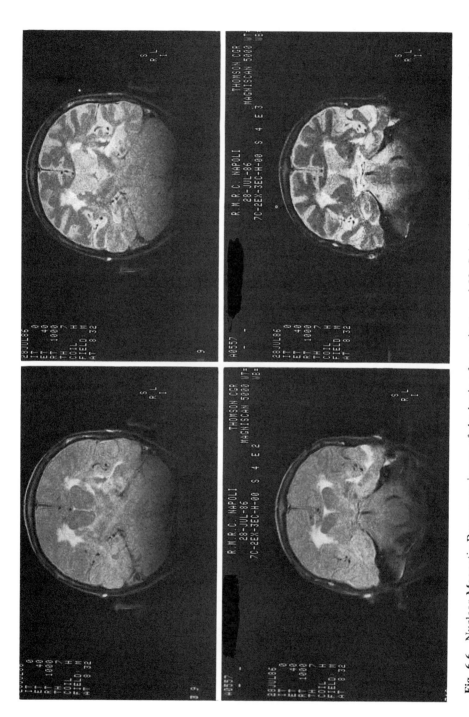

Fig. 6.6 Nuclear Magnetic Resonance image of the brain of a patient aged 80. Spin-echo with multiple echoes technique. Frontal sections. Dilatation of sulci and ventricles with degeneration of the periventricular white matter due to vascular disease.
Courtesy of Dr L. Mossuto Agatiello

REFERENCES

Albert, M., Naeser, M. A., Levine, H. L., and Garvey, A. J. (1984a). Ventricular size in patients with presenile dementia of the Alzheimer type. *Arch. Neurol.*, 41, 1258–1263.

Albert, M., Naeser, M. A., Levine, H. L., and Garvey, A. J. (1984b). CT density numbers in patients with senile dementia of the Alzheimer type. *Arch. Neurol.*, 41, 1264–1269.

Angeleri, F., Provinciali, L., Signorino, M., Piana, C., and Salvolini, U. (1983). Ageing mind, depression and dementia: a neuropsychological, electrophysiological and CT approach to the clinical diagnosis. In A. Cecchini, G. Nappi and A. Arrigo (Eds), *Cerebral Pathology in Old Age.* Pavia: Emiras, pp. 91–102.

Barclay, L., Zemcov, A., Blass, J. P., and McDowell, F. H. (1984). Rapid rate of decline in cerebral blood flow in progressive dementia. In C. Fieschi, G. L. Lenzi and C. Loeb (Eds), *Monograph in Neural Sciences,* vol. 11. Basel: Karger, pp. 107–110.

Benton, A. L., and Sivan, A. B. (1984). Problems and conceptual issues in neuropsychological research in aging and dementia. *J. Clin. Neuropsychol.*, 6, 57–63.

Brinkman, S. D., Sarwar, M., Levin, H. S., and Morris, H. H. (1981). Quantitative indexes of computed tomography in dementia or normal aging. *Neuroradiology*, 138, 89–92.

Bryan, R. N. (1985). Imaging techniques of the aging brain. In C. M. Gaitz and T. Samorajski (Eds). *Aging 2000: Our Health Care Destiny.* New York: Springer-Verlag, pp. 197–201.

Cutler, N. R. (1985). Brain metabolism as measured with positron emission tomography: aging, Alzheimer's disease and Down syndrome. In C. G. Gottfries (Ed.), *Normal Aging, Alzheimer's Disease and Senile Dementia.* Bruxelles: Editions de l'Université, pp. 181–198.

Cutler, N. R., Duara, R., Creasey, H., Grady, C. L., Haxby, J. V., Schapiro, M. B., and Rapoport, S. I. (1984). Brain imaging: aging and dementia. *Ann. Intern. Med.*, 101, 355–369.

Dastur, D. K. (1985). Cerebral blood flow and metabolism in normal human aging, pathological aging, and senile dementia. *J. Cereb. Blood Flow Metabol.*, 5, 1–9.

Davis, S. M., Ackerman, R. H., Correia, J. A., Alpert, N. M., Chang, J., Buonanno, F., Kelly, R. E., Rosner, B., and Taveras, J. M. (1983). Cerebral blood flow and cerebrovascular CO_2 reactivity in stroke-age normal controls. *Neurology*, 33, 391–399.

De Leon, M. J., and George, A. E. (1983). Computed tomography imaging and senile dementia of the Alzheimer type. In R. Mayeux and W. G. Rosen, *Advances in Neurology*, vol. 38. New York: Raven Press, pp. 103–122.

De Leon, M. J., George, A. E., Ferris, S. H., Christmas, D., Gentes, C. I., Miller, J. D., Fowler, J., Reisberg, B., and Wolf, A. P. (1985). CT, PET and NMR brain imaging in aging and Alzheimer's disease. In C. G. Gottfries (Ed.), *Normal Aging,, Alzheimer's Disease and Senile Dementia.* Bruxelles: Editions de l'Université, pp. 199–202.

Dekoninck, W. J., Piraux, A., Uytdenhoef, P., and Jacquay, J. (1982). Relationship between EEG and cerebral blood flow in normal brain aging. *Exp. Brain Res.*, suppl. 5, 208–215.

Duara, R., Margolin, R. A., Robertson-Tchabo, E. A., London, E. D., Schwartz, M., Renfrew, J. W., Koziarz. B. J., Sundaram, M., Grady, C., Moore, A. M., Ingvar, D. H., Sokoloff, L., et al. (1983). Cerebral glucose utilisation, as measured with positron emission tomography in 21 resting healthy men between the ages of 21 and 83 years. *Brain*, 106, 761–775.

Dupui, P., Guell, A., Bessoles, G., Geraud, G., and Bes, A. (1984). Cerebral blood flow in aging. Decrease of hyperfrontal distribution. In C. Fieschi, G. L. Lenzi and C. Loeb (Eds), *Monograph in Neural Sciences,* vol. 11. Basel: Karger, pp. 131–138.

Earnest, M. P., Heaton, R. K., Wilkinson, W. E., and Manke, W. F. (1979). Cortical atrophy, ventricular enlargement and intellectual impairment in the aged. *Neurology*, 29, 1138–1143.

Erkinjuntti, T., Ketonen, L., Sipponen, J., and Sulkava, R. (1985). Nuclear Magnetic Resonance (NMR) imaging in differential diagnosis of Alzheimer's disease (AD) and vascular dementia. *J. Neurol.*, 232 (suppl.), 157.

Ferris, S. H., DeLeon, M. J., Wolf, A. P., George, A. E., Reisberg, B., Brody, J., Gentes,

C., Christmas, D. R., and Fowler, J. S. (1983). Regional metabolism and cognitive deficits in aging and senile dementia. In D. Samuel, S. Algeri, S. Gershon, V. E. Grimm and G. Toffano (Eds), *Aging* vol. 22. New York: Raven Press, pp. 133–142.

Fieschi, C., and Lenzi, G. L. (1983). The aging brain and its metabolic balance: Positron Emission Tomography. Results and prospects. In D. Samuel, S. Algeri, S. Gershon, V. E. Grimm and G. Toffano (Eds), *Aging* vol. 22. New York: Raven Press, pp. 123–131.

Frackowiak, R. S. J., Wise, R. J. S., Gibbs, J. M., Jones, T., and Leenders, N. (1984a). Oxygen extraction in the aging brain. In C. Fieschi, G. L. Lenzi and C. Loeb (Eds), *Monograph in Neural Sciences,* vol. 11. Basel: Karger, pp. 118–122.

Frackowiak, R. S. J., Wise, R. J. S., Gibbs, J. M., and Jones, T. (1984b). Positron Emission Tomographic studies in aging and cerebrovascular disease at Hammersmith Hospital. *Ann. Neurol.* 15(suppl.), S112–S118.

Globus, M., Cooper, G., and Melamed, E. (1984). Reduction in regional blood flow during normal aging is not limited only to elderly subjects. In C. Fieschi, G. L. Lenzi and C. Loeb (Eds), *Monograph in Neural Sciences,* vol. 11. Basel: Karger, pp. 139–143.

Goldstein, S. J., Wekstein, D. R., Kirkpatrick, C., Lee, C., and Markesbery, W. R. (1985). Imaging the centenarian brain. A computed tomographic study. *J. Am. Geriat. Soc.,* 33, 579–584.

Gomori, J. M,., Steiner, I., Melamed, E., and Cooper, G. (1984). The assessment of changes in brain volume using combined linear measurements. A CT-scan study. *Neuroradiology,* 26, 21–24.

Gottstein, U., Held, K., Moller, W., and Berghoff, W. (1970). Utilisation of ketone bodies by the human brain. In J. S. Meyer, M. Reivich and H. Lechner (Eds), *Research on Cerebral Circulation.* Springfield: Charles C. Thomas, pp. 137–145.

Hartmann, A., and Ries, R. (1985). Regional cerebral blood flow change with age in normal humans. *J. Neurol.,* 232 (suppl.), 156.

Herscovitch, P., Gado, M., Mintun, M. A., and Raichle, M. E. (1984). The necessity for correcting for cerebral atrophy in global positron emission tomography measurements. In C. Fieschi, G. L. Lenzi and C. Loeb (Eds), *Monograph in Neural Sciences,* vol. 11. Basel: Karger, pp. 93–97.

Kaszniak, A. W., Garron, D. C., Fox, J. H., Bergen, D., and Huckman, M. (1979). Cerebral atrophy, EEG slowing age, education and cognitive functioning in suspected dementia. *Neurology,* 29, 1273–1279.

Kobayashi, S., Yamaguchi, S., Katsube, T., Kitani, M., Okada, K., and Kitamura, J. (1984). Influence of social environmental factors on cerebral circulation and mental function in the normal aged. In C. Fieschi, G. L. Lenzi and C. Loeb (Eds), *Monograph in Neural Sciences,* vol. 11. Basel: Karger, pp. 163–168.

Kuhl, D. E., Metter, E. J., Riege, W. H., and Hawkins, R. A. (1984). The effect of normal aging on patterns of local cerebral glucose utilization. *Ann. Neurol.,* 15 (suppl.), S133–S137.

Lassen, N. A., and Ingvar, D. H. (1980). Blood flow studies in the aging normal brain and in senile dementia. In L. Amaducci, A. N. Davison and P. Antuono (Eds), *Aging,* vol. 13. New York: Raven Press, pp. 91–98.

Lebrun-Grandié, P., Baron, J. C., Soussaline, F., Loch'h, C., Sastre, J., and Bousser, M. G. (1983). Coupling between regional blood flow and oxygen utilization in the normal human brain. *Arch. Neurol.,* 40, 230–236.

LeMay, M. (1984). Radiological changes in the aging brain and skull. *AJR,* 143, 383–389.

Lenzi, G. L., Frackowiak, R. S. J., Jones, T., Heather, J. D., Lammertsma, A. A., Rhodes, C. G., and Pozzilli, C. (1981). $CMRO_2$ and CBF by oxygen-15 inhalation technique. *Eur. Neurol.,* 20, 285–290.

Lenzi, G. L., and Pantano, P. (1984). Neurological applications of Positron Emission Tomography. *Neurol. Clinics,* 2, 853–871.

Mamo, H., Meric, P., Luft, A., and Seylaz, J. (1983). Hyperfrontal pattern of human cerebral circulation. *Arch. Neurol.,* 40, 626–632.

Masdeau, J., and Aronson, M. (1985). CT findings in early dementia. *Gerontologist*, 25, 82.

McInnes, J. A., Saporta, J. A., and Kelly, R. B. (1985). Neuropsychological performance and CT volumetric measures in the elderly. *Gerontologist*, 25, 87.

Meyer, J. S., and Shaw, T. G. (1984). Cerebral blood flow in aging. In M. L. Albert (Ed.), *Clinical Neurology of Aging*. Oxford: Oxford University Press, pp. 178–196.

Oiwa, K., Shimazu, K., Tamura, N., Hienuki, M., Kim, H. T., Yamamoto, T., and Hamaguchi, K. (1984). Effect of aging on cerebral blood flow autoregulation — with special reference to the role of the prostaglandins. In C. Fieschi, G. L. Lenzi and C. Loeb (Eds), *Monograph in Neural Sciences*, vol. 11. Basel: Karger, pp. 210–215.

Pantano, P., Baron, J. C., Lebrun-Grandié, P., Duquesnoy, N., Bousser, M. G., and Comar, D. (1984a). Effects of normal aging on regional CBF and $CMRO_2$ in humans. In C. Fieschi, G. L. Lenzi and C. Loeb (Eds), *Monograph in Neural Sciences*, vol. 11. Basel: Karger, pp. 123–130.

Pantano, P., Baron, J. C., Lebrun-Grandié, P., Duquesnoy, N., Bousser, M. G., and Comar, D. (1984b). Regional blood flow and oxygen consumption in human aging. *Stroke*, 15, 635–641.

Rapoport, S. I., Duara, R., and Haxby, J. V. (1984). Positron Emission Tomography in normal aging and Alzheimer's disease. *Psychopharmacol. Bull.*, 20, 466–471.

Riege, W. H., Metter, E. J., Kuhl, D. E., and Phelps, M. E. (1985). Brain glucose metabolism and memory functions: age decrease in factor scores. *J. Gerontol.*, 40, 459–467.

Rogers, R. L., Meyer, J. S., Mortel, K. F., Mahurin, R. K., and Thornby, J. (1985). Age-related reductions in cerebral vasomotor reactivity and the law of initial value: a 4-year prospective longitudinal study. *J. Cereb. Blood Flow Metabol.*, 5, 79–85.

Shaw, T. G., Mortel, K. F., Meyer, J. S., Rogers, R. L., Hardenerg, J., and Cutaia, M. M. (1984). Cerebral blood flow changes in benign aging and cerebrovascular disease. *Neurology*, 34, 855–862.

Shinohara, Y., Takagi, S., and Kobatake, K. (1984). Effect of aging on CBF and autoregulation in normal subjects and CVD patients. In C. Fieschi, G. L. Lenzi and C. Loeb (Eds), *Monograph in Neural Sciences*, vol. 11. Basel: Karger, pp. 204–209.

Steiner, I., Gomori, J. M., and Melamed, E. (1985). Progressive brain atrophy during normal aging in man: a quantitative computerized tomography study. *Isr. J. Med. Sci.*, 21, 279–282.

Tachibana, H., Meyer, J. S., Kitagawa, Y., Rogers, R. L., Okayasu, H., and Mortel, K. F. (1984a). Effects of aging on cerebral blood flow in dementia. *J. Am. Geriat. Soc.*, 32, 114–120.

Tachibana, H., Heyer, J. S., Okayasu, H., and Kandula, P. (1984b). Changing topographic patterns of human cerebral blood flow with age measured with Xenon CT. *AJR*, 142, 1027–1034.

Tachibana, H., Meyer, J. S., Kitagawa, Y., Tanahashi, N., Kandula, P., and Rogers, R. L. (1985). Xenon contrast CT-CBF measurements in Parkinsonism and normal aging. *J. Am. Geriat. Soc.*, 33, 413–421.

Takeda, S., and Matsuzawa, T. (1984). Brain atrophy during aging: a quantitative study using Computed Tomography. *J. Am. Geriat. Soc.*, 32, 520–524.

Takeda, S., and Matsuzawa, T. (1985). Age-related change in volumes of the ventricles, cisternae, and sulci: a quantitative study using Computed Tomography. *J. Am. Geriat. Soc.*, 33, 264–268.

Warren, L. R., Butler, R. W., Katholi, C. R., and Halsey jr., J. H. (1985). Age differences in cerebral blood flow during rest and during mental activation measurements with and without monetary incentive. *J. Gerontol.*, 40, 53–59.

Yamamura, H., Ito, M., Kubota, K., and Matsuzawa, T. (1980). Brain atrophy during aging: a quantitative study with computed tomography. *J. Gerontol.*, 35, 492–498.

Zatz, L. M., Jernigan, T. L., and Ahumada, A. J. (1982). Changes on computed cranial tomography with aging: intracranial fluid volume. *J. Neuroradiol.*, 3, 1–11.

Zemcov. A., Barclay, L., and Blass, J. P. (1984). Regional decline of cerebral blood flow with age in cognitively intact subjects. *Neurobiol. Aging*, 5, 1–6.

CHAPTER 7

Volts, hertz, milliseconds

*Brain electrical activity changes only slightly with age in spite of the transforma-
tion taking place in its cytoarchitecture. The changes in dementia are much more
pronounced.*

The electrical activity of the brain provides us with on-line, real-time access to the
substrate of mental processes. With a time resolution of milliseconds, it reveals
the fleeting dynamics of mental activity to which imaging techniques like PET,
NMR and CBF are blind. We shall consider the contribution of electrophysiological studies under two headings. First, electroencephalography which is concerned
with the on-going electrical activity of the brain, and then evoked potentials which
assess the responsiveness of particular sensory and perceptual system.

ELECTROENCEPHALOGRAPHY (EEG)

The electrical activity of the human brain was discovered by Berger in 1929, but
systematic studies of age-related changes in the EEG were not published until the
1950s (Mundy-Castle et al., 1954): there is a significant difference in the frequency
of alpha rhythm in the aged, 10.32 Hz in a young control group and 9.39 Hz in
subjects with an average age of 75 years. In the EEG traces of the normal aged
these authors find that 24% have anomalies of various types, but in patients with

signs of deterioration the proportion goes up to 54%. Thus the background activity of the EEG in the elderly shows characteristics that would be abnormal, if they were found in a young population (Silverman et al., 1955). In a subsequent study (Obrist et al. 1963), the alpha frequency of a healthy aged group was found to have an average value of 9.16 Hz, while that of deteriorated subjects is around 8 Hz. Correlation of frequency with cerebral blood flow and brain metabolism was found only in the deteriorated subjects, indicating that age is not responsible for EEG alterations. In the same study a prevalence of fast beta activity is described as a characteristic of the aging process, with a decrease after 80. According to research into demographic factors influencing the EEG of the elderly, the beta has a higher incidence in lower income classes, especially in women (Wang and Busse, 1969). Furthermore, women have a more accelerated alpha frequency than men. Beta activity is found in the tracings of the very old, over 100 years. In these subjects average alpha rhythm has been reported to have a frequency of 8.62 Hz, if those with 'generalized arteriosclerosis' are discounted. In one 105 year old subject the alpha frequency was still 9 Hz. The authors of this study propose that no significant changes occur in the EEG of normal subjects after the age of 80 (Hubbard et al., 1976).

Spectral analysis of the EEG has permitted us to verify and extend many of these findings (Giaquinto, 1980). This type of analysis transforms the data from the time domain to the frequency domain (Figs. 7.1 and 7.2). In place of many pages of EEG traces we obtain a Cartesian diagram with the power on the Y-axis and the frequency on the X-axis. Spectral analysis relies on the Fast Fourier Transform (FFT) to calculate the power of the signal in each of the frequency bands of which it is composed.

The first study of this type applied to the aged showed a slight increase in relative power in the slow delta and theta band, a slight decrease in the alpha and an increase in the faster activity beta-2, which spans the frequencies 30 to 40 Hz (Roubicek, 1977). The presence of these rhythms in the aged (Fig. 7.3) is considered to be a favourable sign by Roubicek, as evidenced by their correlation with good mental capacity. A drop of the beta in demented subjects confirms this view (Coben et al., 1983; Giaquinto and Nolfe, 1986).

A factor analysis has been carried out on 619 normal subjects of different ages from 20 to 95 years, including the frequency of five EEG bands (Matejcek, 1980). In a factor which is age-related, the variable age has the highest loading followed by the dominant alpha frequency, which is negatively correlated with age.

The calculation of the correlation coefficient between age and EEG frequencies provides a number of significant effects (Tables 7.1 and 7.2). Alpha frequency is negatively correlated with age, while the theta frequency is positively correlated. A significant correlation is found between age and relative power in the theta band, particularly in those areas which are vulnerable to anatomical changes during the aging process.

A reduced response to hyperventilation and to intermittent light stimulation has been noticed along with the slowing of the alpha rhythm (Hughes and Cayaffa, 1977). A reduced sensitivity to hyperventilation in the elderly has not confirmed by others (Soininen et al., 1982), who have found a positive response in 66% of

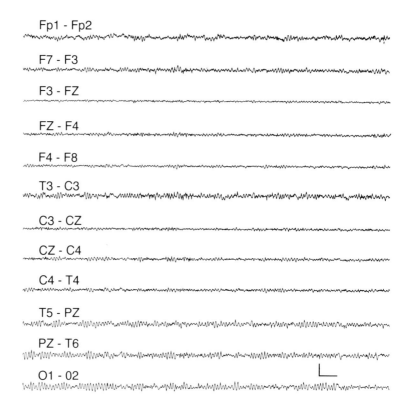

Fp1 - Fp2

F7 - F3

F3 - FZ

FZ - F4

F4 - F8

T3 - C3

C3 - CZ

CZ - C4

C4 - T4

T5 - PZ

PZ - T6

O1 - 02

Fig. 7.1   EEG of a man aged 80. It shows that the background activity can be regular without pathological transients even at that age. Calibration: 1 sec, 50μV

cases. Perhaps the results of hyperventilation depend on ventilation capacity rather than altered brain reactivity. For example, more recent research found a positive response to hyperventilation in the aged in only 26% of the cases studied (Torres et al., 1983). Alpha rhythm reactivity also decreases with age. The ratio of power in the alpha band with eyes open to that with eye closed drops linearly with age (Duffy et al., 1984a,b). The correlation coefficient is 0.434, significant at $p<0.001$.

Interestingly enough, the concept of the alpha deceleration during aging has been questioned by recent investigators, along with the idea of a general decline in cognitive abilities. Studies conducted on perfectly healthy aged subjects fail to confirm the slowing of EEG frequencies. In one of these investigations (Katz and Horowitz, 1982) a high alpha frequency is found (i.e. 9.8 Hz) in subjects aged 70. Duffy et al. (1984a,b) suggest that whether slowing is found depends on the selection of subjects. In those who remain healthy and mentally alert there is no change in alpha frequency and little decline in alpha power. We have compared a group of the aged with a group of younger subjects between 40 and 60 and found

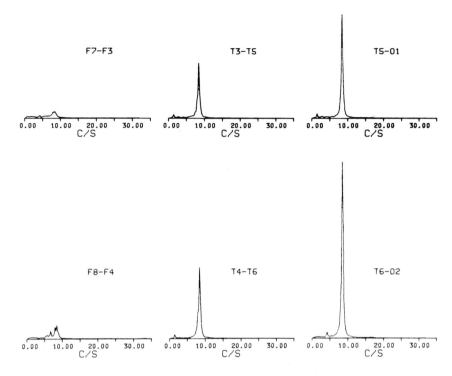

Fig. 7.2 Power spectra of the EEG of a normal 70-year-old subject. Upper row: left hemisphere. Lower row: right hemisphere. From left to right: frontal, temporal and occipital leads. Each spectrum displays a dominant alpha peak, which is higher in occipital leads

no significant differences (Giaquinto and Nolfe, 1986). Much of the literature on this topic is devoted to activity in the occipital region which has the highest alpha rhythm. However, it is important to consider regional differences, because frontal, temporal, and parietal areas are known to undergo greater morphological change than the occipital cortex during aging. In a group of healthy subjects ($N=47$, mean age 71 years) who were not receiving any medical treatment and who did not use hypnotics, we found a high degree of symmetry and a typical topographic distribution of the EEG in line with other investigators (Visser et al., 1985). The frequency of alpha rhythm over left and right hemispheres was remarkably similar at homotopic points, namely 9.07 Hz and 9.07 Hz in the frontal areas, 9.16 Hz and 9.15 Hz in the temporal areas, 9.26 Hz and 9.29 Hz in the occipital areas. The power in the five bands of the spectrum is shown in Figs. 7.4, 7.5 and in Tables 7.3 and 7.4. The pattern shows the low amplitude of alpha activity in anterior regions and its maximum values posteriorly which is characteristic of the EEG in all normal adults. The data so far discussed reveal a continuum in the EEG from youth, through middle life to old age. If there is any slowing of

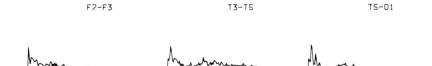

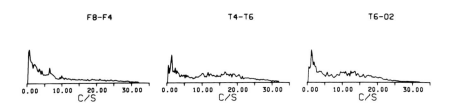

Fig. 7.3 Power spectra from the EEG of a normal 70-year-old subject. The visual EEG is of the beta-dominant variant. Also in this case, the frequency distribution is symmetrical on both sides

Table 7.1 Values of the correlation coefficient between age and mean weighted frequency. Class of age: 60–80 years

Derivation	delta	theta	alpha	beta-1	beta-2
F3-F7 (left frontal)	−.198	.492**	−.376*	−.04	−.391*
F4-F8 (right frontal)	.115	.416*	−.385*	.295	−.273
T3-T5 (left middle temporal)	−.022	.325	−.407*	−.02	−.034
T4-T6 (right middle temporal)	.08	.221	−.389*	−.21	−.03
T5-O1 (left temporo-occipital)	−.130	.353*	−.303	−.23	.181
T6-O2 (right temporo-occipital)	.021	.447*	−.351	−.31	.131

* P<.05
**P<.01

Table 7.2   Values of the correlation coefficient between age and relative activity. Class of
age: 60–80 years. N=32 alpha dominant subjects

Derivation	delta	theta	alpha	beta-1	beta-2
F3-F7 (left frontal)	.244	.08	−.146	−.203	−.405*
F4-F8 (right frontal)	−.1	.202	−.045	−.103	−.01
T3-T5 (left middle temporal)	.047	.436*	−.091	−.272	−.138
T4-T6 (right middle temporal)	.097	.466**	−.238	−.243	−.013
T5-O1 (left temporo-occipital)	.185	.464**	−.244	−.140	−.153
T6-O2 (right temporo-occipital)	.229	.444*	−.177	−.258	−.241

* P<.05
**P<.01

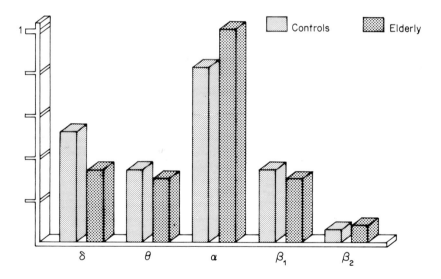

Fig. 7.4   T3-T5 lead. Mean frequency bands from 48 normal elderly subjects (mean
age 71). Controls are represented by 20 middle-aged normal subjects (mean age 55).
Differences are not significant

alpha activity, it stabilizes after 80, and many researchers deny that it occurs at all
in healthy, mentally active subjects. There are some differences in age-related
changes in other parts of the spectrum, however. Using spectral analysis our data

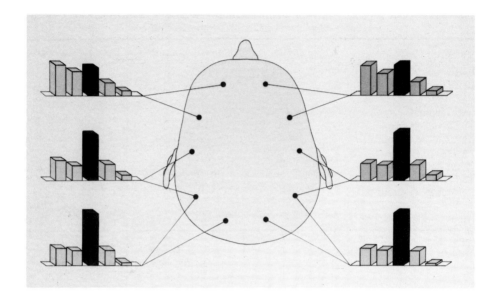

Fig. 7.5 Automatic analysis of the EEG. Distribution on the scalp of the five frequency bands. For each lead, the central block represents the alpha band, the low-frequency bands (delta and theta) are on the left and the high-frequency bands (beta-1 and beta-2) are on the right. This figure cumulates power spectra from 48 normal elderly subjects

(Fig. 7.6) confirm the early finding of Wang and Busse (1969) which were obtained by measurement of the raw EEG. With increasing age, beta activity holds up more strongly in women, while the low frequency delta activity begins to show more strongly in men. This accords with the fact that men are affected sooner by aging than women, since slow frequencies are associated with impairment of cognitive performance.

EEG anomalies are present in about a third of all subjects over 65, but in as many as 94% of those with Alzheimer's dementia the figures vary somewhat from study to study. This promises to provide us with a much clearer discrimination between normal aging and dementia than was possible with any of the morphological or molecular techniques we considered earlier in this book. Before we can follow this lead it is necessary to consider what is meant by a normal EEG.

Guggenheim and Karbowski (1979) report that only 39 (22.9%) out of 170 healthy subjects aged 40 to 60 had an EEG entirely free from 'anomalies' of one type or another. These middle-aged subjects had a mean alpha frequency of 9.9 Hz but a range of 8.6 to 11.2 Hz. Ten per cent had accentuated theta activity (see Table 7.5). Such left temporal anomalies are often seen in the normal aged. Indeed many of the abnormalities which occur in the elderly were also present in this group of middle-aged normals. Focal abnormalities are more common in patients with neurological problems than in the normal aged or in healthy young

Table 7.3 Percentiles of cumulative distribution of relative activity in a normal elderly group

Channel	EEG band	P_{50}	P_{90}
F3F7	delta	25.2	45.2
	theta	15.7	35.4
	alpha	20.4	40.2
	beta-1	10.1	22.1
	beta-2	3.1	7.0
T3T5	delta	10.6	35.1
	theta	10.4	25.1
	alpha	40.2	70.2
	beta-1	12.0	30.0
	beta-2	1.4	11.1
T5O1	delta	10.3	30.2
	theta	10.4	25.0
	alpha	50.1	75.3
	beta-1	10.1	26.0
	beta-2	2.0	4.0
F4F8	delta	25.2	45.1
	theta	15.7	35.1
	alpha	25.1	40.3
	beta-1	12.0	20.0
	beta-2	3.1	7.2
T4T6	delta	10.0	30.6
	theta	10.3	35.1
	alpha	40.1	75.0
	beta-1	10.6	29.7
	beta-2	1.3	11.1
T6O2	delta	10.3	30.3
	theta	10.3	20.6
	alpha	50.0	75.2
	beta-1	12.0	28.1
	beta-2	1.5	4.1

subjects, and age is not an important factor in their occurrence in subjects under 64 (Matousek et al., 1967). We agree with other authors (including Obrist et al., 1963; Kooi et al., 1964; Sokoloff, 1966; Kazis et al., 1982) that general and focal abnormalities are due to slight pathological alterations that can occur at any age, although they are more frequent in older people. It is difficult to explain the prevalence of focal slow activity in the left temporal area (see Busse, 1983) or in the right hemisphere, in spite of a good maintenance of the electrical activity in the aged brain (Duffy et al., 1984a). It follows that the presence of some anomalies in the EEG is not in itself evidence of clinically significant cerebral malfunction.

Nevertheless, as a group, demented subjects are distinguished by the propor-

Table 7.4 Percentiles of cumulative distribution of weighted mean frequency in the elderly group

Channel	EEG band	P_{50}	P_{90}
F3F7	delta	1.28	1.54
	theta	5.05	5.52
	alpha	9.01	9.28
	beta-1	16.00	16.51
	beta-2	25.76	26.26
T3T5	delta	1.29	1.53
	theta	5.27	5.77
	alpha	9.03	9.75
	beta-1	15.76	16.51
	beta-2	25.51	26.25
T5O1	delta	1.30	1.54
	theta	5.27	5.75
	alpha	9.26	9.77
	beta-1	15.50	16.25
	beta-2	25.52	26.26
F4F8	delta	1.28	1.53
	theta	5.27	5.54
	alpha	9.01	9.28
	beta-1	15.78	16.76
	beta-2	25.52	26.26
T4T6	delta	1.9	1.55
	theta	5.27	5.54
	alpha	9.25	9.52
	beta-1	15.76	16.50
	beta-2	25.52	26.50
T6O2	delta	1.29	1.54
	theta	5.27	5.75
	alpha	9.26	9.77
	beta-1	15.28	15.78
	beta-2	25.51	26.01

tion who show abnormalities. Torres et al. (1983), for example, found anomalies in 52% of normal elderly subjects but in 82% of patients with dementia. This difference is striking even though the figure of 52% for the normal elderly is somewhat higher than is usually reported.

Discrimination of the normal elderly from demented subjects improves if we examine the EEG quantitatively. Spectral analysis reveals that delta and theta activity increase in power in dementia, at the expense of alpha and beta activity (Penttila et al., 1985; Visser et al., 1985; Giaquinto and Nolfe, 1986).

Alpha rhythm flattens out in the early stages of dementia (Coben et al., 1983; Ono et al., 1982) to be replaced by slow diffuse rhythms with eventual paroxysms. The EEG changes appear to be more helpful in detecting cases of Alzheimer's

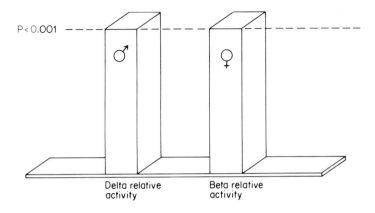

Fig. 7.6 Significant sex-linked differences in the elderly. Compared with men, women have less delta and more beta frequency

Table 7.5 Percentage of abnormal EEG tracings in normal elderly and demented subjects

Reference	Normal	Demented
Mundy-Castle et al. (1954)	24%	54%
Gerson and Chat (1967)	21%	89%
Soininen et al. (1982)	29%	94%
Torres et al. (1983)	52%	82%

dementia than CT scans, because the changes occur so early in the disease (Angeleri et al., 1983). This is supported by a recent study (Penttila et al., 1985) which shows that the changes mainly affect the percentage power of the theta band, the ratio of powers in the alpha and theta bands and the mean frequency (range 1.46–20.02 Hz). There appears to be no close relationship between the seriousness of the disease and the extent of the EEG damage (Gordon and Sim, 1967). In doubtful cases it is advisable to repeat the recording after three months and to compare the spectra. Alpha frequency changes little from test to test at least among the young subjects (Gasser et al., 1985) and a reduction in predominant frequency is therefore meaningful. A single EEG recording may yield a false negative diagnosis (Liston, 1979), although according to other authors (Gordon and Sim, 1967), the tracing is always pathological in Alzheimer's dementia. In this it is distinguished from Pick's dementia. Tasks involving both resting EEG and evoked response measures discriminated cognitively impaired elderly subjects from a control group matched for sex, race, age and education with 82% accuracy (John et al., 1977).

No relationship has been so far established between EEG changes and CT scan data. No correlation was found between the prevalence of EEG abnormalities and the degree of brain atrophy, as measured by the distance between the most lateral points of the frontal horns and of the white matter of the third ventricle (Stefoski et al., 1976) nor between EEG abnormalities and relationships between parenchyma and fluid spaces (Gastaut et al., 1980). Although there was no relationship between EEG variables and CT scan or age in this study, EEG changes were found to correlate with mental decline. On the other hand, ventricular volume was found to correlate with age but not with mental state. The relationship between EEG frequency and cognitive impairment but not between EEG and signs of physical atrophy, like ventricular dilatation, has been confirmed by others (Roberts et al., 1978; Angeleri et al., 1983). A similar conclusion was reached by Kaszniak et al. (1979) in an investigation which used EEG, CT scan and neuropsychological tests on 78 subjects with suspected deterioration but without focal neurological signs of other evident organic damage. The conclusion from this study is that the EEG is a more valuable indicator of cognitive impairment than morphology and that the slowing of its dominant frequency is the important measure.

To summarize, the EEG in elderly people in good mental and physical health maintains the same general characteristics as that of young controls. Spectral analysis shows that the frequency and the power of the alpha rhythm maintains its topographic distribution on the scalp with higher values over the occipital areas. There are no significant left–right asymmetries in the resting EEG at least in the power spectrum. There is a good agreement among authors on the value of alpha frequency in the elderly both with visual inspection and automatic analysis. Any slowing of this rhythm in the normal aged is certainly not greater than 1 Hz (Table 7.6).

The final topic of this section deals with the intriguing problem of the relationship between EEG and mental activity. Relatively little work has been done on this topic in the elderly, chiefly because the Wechsler Adult Intelligence Scale (WAIS) has proved so useful in assessing mental abilities directly even though it was not designed for the elderly population. In general, WAIS scores are relatively stable over time. In a group of 32 healthy subjects who received both EEG and WAIS tasks on two occasions, more than three years apart, there were no significant changes in the WAIS assessments (Wang et al., 1974). On this evidence Gastaut (1974) expressed the view that the EEG changes, especially in the alpha rhythm, are unrelated to psychological functions.

Nevertheless, the concept that resting EEG monitors the integrity of the underlying cortex has encouraged other investigators to seek relationships with cognitive functions in the elderly. Their task has been greatly assisted by the advent of computerized EEG analysis. A correlation matrix between EEG and psychological variables reveals a number of low but nevertheless significant coefficients, indicating vigilance affects both EEG frequencies and perceptual and mental activity (Ott et al., 1982). In a population of active and bright elderly

Table 7.6 Alpha mean frequency in normal elderly subjects

Reference	Alpha frequency
Mundy-Castle et al. (1954)	9.39
Obrist et al. (1963)	9.16
Otomo (1966)	9.47
Wang and Busse (1969)	9.08 (men)
	9.44 (women)
Harner (1975)	9.40
Hubbard et al. (1976)	8.56*
Hughes and Cayaffa (1977)	9.00**
Matejcek (1980)	8.75†
Soininen et al. (1982)	9.03
Katz and Horowitz (1982)	9.80
Torres et al. (1983)	9.70
Giaquinto and Nolfe (1986)	9.46‡
Visser et al. (1985)	9.60

*data from centenarians
**approximated values
†value from curve
‡occipital values

women EEG power in the so called sigma band (13.2–14.8 Hz) recorded from parietal lobes is associated with a high score on the WAIS and other tests of cognitive ability (Patterson et al., 1983). Consistent correlations also exist between bilateral theta activity and Bender Gestalt copying, between Wechsler Memory Scale, mental control and bilateral slow alpha activity.

It is important to distinguish between studies like those of Ott et al. (1982) and Patterson et al. (1983) in which test scores are correlated with features of the EEG recorded at rest and studies in which the EEG is recorded during mental activity itself. Typically, the EEG is recorded during the performance of tasks. Our own observations confirm, within certain limits, the correlation of EEG data with neurophysiological findings including reaction times, tachistoscopy and memory tasks. The results are shown in Table 7.7. It is a familiar problem in statistics that multiple tests throw up 'significant' values at a frequency specified by the confidence limit even when the data are random. In our study more of the correlations reached the confidence limit than would be expected by chance alone indicating that the relationship between EEG and behavioural measures is genuine.

Sleep

Numerous studies of sleep in the elderly have appeared in the literature (see Dement et al., 1982). In this section we consider the main findings. While awake, the elderly subject undergoes brief periods of EEG deceleration characterized by frequencies between 1 and 7 Hz and patterns corresponding to 'microsleeps'. These microsleeps are more frequent in elderly people living in conditions of poor

Table 7.7   Correlations: EEG—neuropsychological tests

6 channels	F3-F7, T3-T5, T5-O1; F4-F8, T4-T6, T6-O1
5 spectral bands	delta, theta, alpha, beta-1, beta-2
2 spectral parameters	mean frequency, relative power
7 tests	words and numbers tachistoscopy
	pattern recognition
	choice reaction time
	free recall
	block tapping
	delayed recall

Total number of possible correlation coefficients: $6 \times 5 \times 2 \times 7 = 420$
Significant correlation coefficients: 33 at 0.05 level of significance
Correlation coefficients due to chance: 21

stimulation. In the first sleep stages delta activity (0.2–4 Hz) slows down, as the quantity of high frequency and low voltage activity diminishes. In the REM stage, when ocular movements occur, delta, theta and sometimes alpha appear, which are not usually present in the REM sleep of younger people. REM is therefore less uniform than normal. Smith et al. (1977) have examined the occurrence of spindles during sleep. Spindles are specific graphic elements of EEG traces composed of characteristic sinusoid activity of low amplitude and short duration that are prevalent on the central and frontal regions. Spindles are less common in elderly people than in young controls, aged between 25 and 34. However, change occurs before old age because their incidence is not different from that of 45–53 year olds (Smith et al., 1977). This seems to be another argument in favour of a 'continuum' between young and old, mathematically a function with a very weak negative derivative. The positive occipital sharp transients of sleep are present until the 70s. As has recently been repeated, they are not restricted to much younger age groups (Wright and Gilmore, 1985). These potentials are, however, missing in very abnormal EEG tracings.

Older people spend more time in bed, whether or not they are attempting to sleep or taking short naps. The increasing amount of time spent in bed is not associated with more sleep. In the aged the period of total sleep starting from the main day sleep is too variable, while the actual sleeping time is the same or less, not calculating the time spent in bed in wakefulness. The aged are prone to reawakening after first falling asleep, and the time to fall asleep is increased or unchanged compared to that in young adulthood. It is still unclear whether the quality of sleep is reduced in the aged. The most reliable EEG data are the absolute and relative reduction of stage 4 sleep, which in 25% of the older population is missing (Prinz et al., 1982). The duration of REM sleep diminishes, yet it still occurs to some extent even at a very advanced age. When REM sleep diminishes, the associated physiological activities are also reduced, including myoclonus, heart rate and breathing irregularities, increased blood flow and penis erection. REM sleep unusually tends to be concentrated in the first part of the night (Figs. 7.7 and 7.8), but there is a number of interesting differences. Women have more continuous sleep, a higher percentage of stage 3 and greater REM activity (Reynolds et al., 1985). Early reawakenings are more frequent in both young and older men, while the sensation of feeling worse in the morning than in the evening diminishes with age, perhaps due to evening discomforts experienced by older people (Abe and Suzuki, 1985).

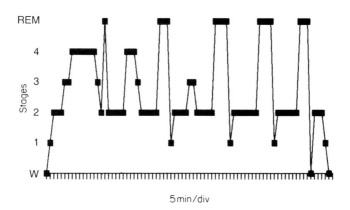

Fig. 7.7 'Sleep profile from a young volunteer. Five REM episodes have occurred throughout the night, with quite regular onset

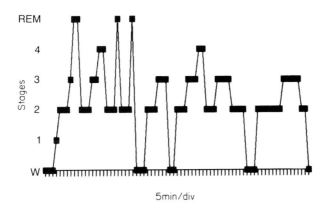

Fig. 7.8 Sleep profile from a normal 70-year-old subject. REM episodes are few and mainly concentrated in the first hours. The stage 4 is sparse

Sleep deprivation is more keenly felt in younger people but on objective measures the performance decrement is greater in the elderly, as measured on persistency tasks, such as the localization of targets embedded in noise or simple tasks of arithmetic (Webb, 1985).

Following artificial awakenings, elderly subjects perform slightly less well than the young on tests of recall. Dream narration does not appear to be much impaired, while the visual imageries of dreams are reduced (Fein et al., 1985).

The incidence of sleep apnoea is said to be high among the aged, although recent research indicates that it is less common than sometimes stated. Only 26% of an aged population experience three or more episodes of apnoea per night, compared to 8% of a young control group (Bixler et al., 1985). Risk factors are obesity, hypertension, mental deterioration and chronic obstruction in the air passage. Snoring increases with age: 60% of males snore after 60 years of age. Snoring is not simply an inconvenience for others; it is another risk factor for apnoea itself. Sleep apnoea is very rare at high altitude, presumably due to the reduced atmospheric pressure. In the longeval community of Vilcabamba, mentioned in Chapter 2, it occurs with a much lower incidence compared with the general population (Okudaira et al., 1983).

The sleep of the aged is influenced by the excessive time spent in bed, by lack of stimulation, retirement and by hospitalization. In some institutions unqualified geriatric workers administer too many sedatives, and isolate and restrain those who disturb the peace of the unit during the night (Dement et al., 1982).

EVOKED POTENTIALS

Visual evoked potential (VEP)

The use of the evoked response technique in the study of aging is relatively recent. One of the pioneering studies in this field (Straumanis et al., 1965) examined the potentials evoked by flashes of light in the normal elderly, in senile patients and in young controls. The greatest difference was found between the young and the old, the early components having a longer latency and a higher amplitude in the aged subjects. The senile patients differed from the normal elderly in the later components, which occurred at greater latency and reduced amplitude. Moreover, interhemispheric covariance in the VEP is less in deteriorated subjects discriminating them from the normal elderly even more clearly than changes in the spectrum of the ongoing EEG (Gerson et al., 1976). A scatter diagram of interhemispheric covariance against psychometric evaluation separates the normal elderly and the senile demented into fairly distinct groups. The latency and amplitude of the visual evoked response is thought to discriminate between the two groups more effectively than the somatosensory potential (SEP). These parameters also show a good correlation with some subtests of the WAIS (Boening, 1980). Recent VEP studies have employed pattern reversal stimulation instead of stroboscopic flashes. Typically the black and white squares of a chequer-board are interchanged at a certain frequency.

The pattern reversal potential consists of a negative peak, N1, at about 75 msec, followed by a positive peak, P1, with a latency of about 100 msec. These components had mean values of 73.3 msec and 97.8 msec in subjects varying in age from 18 to 79 years. The graph of latency against age for individual subjects shows that the latency of N1 and P1 increases with age. This has been attributed to slower conduction along the optical nerve fibres (Celesia and Daly, 1977). A reduction in the number of fibres in the optic nerve has been mentioned in Chapter 4, but we shall see later that factors other than changes in peripheral pathways must be responsible for the slowing of the evoked potentials and cognitive functions. The latency distribution for N1 and P1 indicates an average lengthening of 6 msec between 30 and 70 years old, equivalent to a delay of 1.5 msec decade. These changes have been confirmed by Snyder et al. (1981) who also show that the amplitudes of these components remain stable. Indeed, in healthy individuals the only change in amplitude occurs between infancy and adolescence.

Greater changes are found in the late components. The most reliable marker is the P2 peak evoked by flashes. The latency covaries with age even after correction for the effects of pupillary variations, which cause a 0.38 log retinal illuminance decrease in the aged, as the average pupil diameter goes from 4.9 mm at 20 years of age to 3.15 at 70 (Wright et al., 1985). In the case of the pattern reversal VEP too, the late peaks (N130, P165, P220) are delayed and their amplitude increases (Visser et al., 1985). Other authors confirm the usefulness of the VEP in the correct identification of Alzheimer's dementia, emphasizing the behaviour of more stable early peaks (Wright et al., 1984; Harding et al., 1985). In later life there may be a reduction of the inhibitory processes of the visual system which enhances the contrast at contours. It has been suggested that this reduction of inhibition is due to the reduction of the central monoamines and not to peripheral defects (Dustman et al., 1981). Such effects may be responsible for the changing latency of VEP components and increasing amplitude at least of the late components.

Somatosensory evoked potential (SEP)

In the field of somatosensory evoked potentials interindividual variability is minimized by measuring the interpeak latencies, that is to say time intervals between successive peaks (Hume et al., 1982). The SEP to stimulation of the median nerve contains a negative peak at approximately 14 msec in recordings from the neck and 20 msec in recordings from the scalp, thus providing a measure of about 6 msec for central conduction time. Central conduction time is independent of changes in peripheral conduction velocity (Buchtal and Rosenfalck, 1966). Recent calculations indicate a peripheral slowing of 2 m/sec/decade. In the 15–24 age group the sensory and motor conduction velocity of the cutaneous nerve is 70 m/sec and in the 65–74 age band the value is 58 m/sec (Trojaborg, 1976).

In responses to median and tibial nerve stimulation, increases of SEP latencies of respectively 0.015 and 0.08 msec/yr have been found as well as decreases in the speed of motor and sensory conduction (Dorfman and Bosley, 1979). Spinal conduction stays stable until the 50s and then declines at rate of 0.78 m/sec/year. These data indicate that peripheral conduction is of great importance in many of the physical problems of old age including those of balance and locomotion. We shall look at age-dependent changes in the peripheral nervous system and in muscle in Chapter 9.

The changes in sensory pathways have also been studied by Desmedt and Cheron (1980). They report that, although propagation delay in the first order afferent neurons increases by 16 msec, there are no such changes along the spinal cord and up to the generation of the cortical potential. On the other hand, an increase in the latency of the early components in the SEP after the fourth decade has been recently described. The variations among the observations appear to depend somewhat on the techniques employed. Age related changes in the SEP are more evident in men than women (Allison et al., 1984) in addition to the fact that the latencies of N20 and P25 are about 0.40 msec shorter in women than men (Simpson and Erwin, 1983). Only P25 increases in latency with age, though not linearly. Since it is believed that N20 and P25 are generated in different cortical areas, respectively areas 3b and 1 of Brodmann, the authors infer that aging is not uniform throughout the cortex. A similar conclusion can be drawn from histological studies as we saw in Chapter 4.

Acoustic evoked potential (AEP)

Factors contributing to variations in the AEP were the subject of early studies in the evoked response literature (Marsh and Thompson, 1972). Stimulus parameters are particularly important in determining the latencies of individual components (Pfefferbaum et al., 1979). The study in which AEPs from young and old women are compared found the greatest differences in latency (40 msec) in the late AEP components recorded from frontal electrodes using a high stimulus intensity (90 dB). Increasing stimulus intensity was accompanied by decreasing latency and increasing amplitude in these components in both groups of subjects. Subsequent studies (Pfefferbaum et al., 1980a and b) confirmed the latency increase of the late components in the older subjects and revealed a widened P2 component and altered scalp distribution of P3. No differences were found in the early components such as N1, which remains at about 100 msec. The stability claimed for the latency of early AEP components throughout life is not altogether supported by observations of the auditory potentials of the brain stem (BAEP = brain stem auditory evoked potential, or BSEP = brain stem evoked potentials). The latency in BAEP peaks is delayed in people of advanced age, indeed aging is the only physiological factor which slows them; on the other hand, the interpeak latencies do not vary (Rowe, 1978; Rossini et al., 1979; Jerger and Hall, 1980; Allison et al., 1984). Incidentally, there are sex differences in the BAEPs. The latencies of waves I and VII are shorter in women in whom there are also shorter interpeak delays and some peaks have higher amplitudes.

P3 response

The P3 or P300 response is a late component of evoked responses, generated when subjects have to discriminate different stimulus events. Peaks N2 and P3 are delayed in the aged by 32 msec and 44–45 msec, respectively. The latency of P3 continues to increase during advanced age by 1.6 msec/yr (Beck et al., 1980). The various peaks of an evoked response are not equivalent from a neuropsychological standpoint. If a stimulus which carries particular information is sent to the subject, the early components (both N1 and the following P2) increase in amplitude if the information is to be actively processed for a decision. Experiments (for reasons of brevity not treated here in detail) show that a subsequent N2 covaries with the reaction times. P3 on the other hand is like an electric equivalent of the close of the cognitive operation, a resetting for new operations (Fig. 7.9).

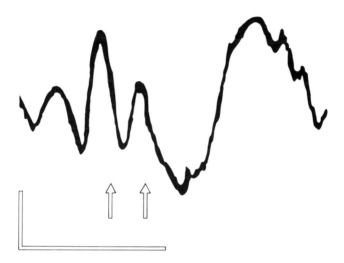

Fig. 7.9   P3 response induced during a visual discrimination task in a normal 65-year-old. Calibration: 300 msec, 5μV. The left arrow indicates the mean simple reaction time in this subject. The right arrow indicates the mean choice reaction time. The P3 is considered as the resetting of a cognitive state

The P3 response is therefore a cognitive potential related to discrimination more than to the physical characteristics of the stimulus. In elderly subjects the amplitude of P3 is reduced, and thus there is an age-change in this physiological correlate of cognitive activity. Elderly people find it relatively difficult to pass from a test which involves attention divided by interference to a test requiring undivided attention. This deficit in sustained attention is accompanied by a reduction in the amplitude of P3 recorded from central and parietal areas in the elderly. Over frontal regions, however, P3 maintains its amplitude revealing the persistence of other orientation mechanisms in the aged (Tecce et al., 1982). The reduction in P3 is confirmed by other authors (Ford et al., 1979; Pfefferbaum et al., 1980a and 1984) who also report a parallel increase in its latency in associated motor tasks, such as reaction time. In experiments of this kind difficulty can be manipulated. For example, if the subject has to decide whether a picture shown to him was included among samples presented a second earlier, the number of samples can be varied. When the number of samples increases from one to four,

P3 is delayed by 85 msec in the young but 165 msec in the elderly, though the difference did not achieve statistical significance. Over the life span the latency increase of the P3 is not linear, accelerating after 45 years of age from 0.53 to 3.14 msec/yr (Brown et al., 1983). According to other authors (Mullis et al., 1985; Polich et al., 1985) the latency of the P3 during the course of life may be represented by a U-shaped function, with its minimum around the third decade. Moreover, this research suggested that the potential has its maximum over anterior regions of the scalp in the elderly whereas in children the peak is located more posteriorly. On the other hand, in more recent research a posterior shift in P3 is seen, being mainly located in the parietal central vertex with a positive correlation with age (Duffy et al., 1984a). It is worth noting that there are substantial differences in the P3 latency and amplitude between the normal aged population and patients with brain atrophy as revealed by CT scan (Angeleri et al., 1983).

P3 latency is a potentially useful measure in differentiating dementia from pseudo-dementia. In a study of 26 normal subjects and 7 depressed ones, no one was misclassified as demented, while 10 out of 18 demented cases were correctly classified (Brown et al., 1982). The authors argue that P3 latency normally increases at a rate of 2.77 msec/yr, but is longer in the demented than in age-matched controls, by at least two standard deviations.

Other studies confirm the longer latency in dementia but indicate a yearly increase in latency, for example 1.2 msec (Neshige et al., 1985). Interestingly enough, in view of the claimed role of the cholinergic system in dementia in some patients P3 latency became shorter following the administration of the anti-cholinesterase physostigmine.

Differences between the aged and controls are therefore more evident when the so-called cognitive potentials are measured under conditions in which the subject is not a passive observer but must make decisions. If in a semantic task the last word of a sequence is illogical, a negative deflection, called by its latency N400, is recorded from the scalp. Examples of this type of sequence are: 'all the birds are trees' and 'dog, cat, bear, mole, grape'. The negative deflection to such semantic incongruity is delayed by up to 90 msec in elderly subjects (Harbin et al., 1984). If, on the other hand, the subject has to recognize whether the fifth word is identical to one of the previous words, the latency is reduced in both aged subjects and in the controls, though the response is still later in the aged subjects.

Before closing this topic it is worth noting that subtle differences between aged and control subjects can be influenced by experimental conditions. In contrast with a former study (Beck et al., 1980) where the P3 delay was found to increase at the rate of 0.8 msec/yr in those aged 28–63 and by 1.6 msec between 63 and 79, one of the authors found no changes in the P3 latency with aging using different procedures (Podlesny and Dustman, 1982).

The events following P3 generally called 'late activity' also change in the aged. When subjects undertake tasks in which they must withhold some responses there is a significant increase in negative mean amplitude of these 'sustained' potentials when they operate and a higher positivity when they hold back (Podlesny et al.,

1984). P300, N400 and late activity are of particular interest in studies of aging because they appear to monitor the substrate of cognitive as opposed to sensory processes and it is the former which is impaired especially in dementia. However, these phenomena are still at the stage of taxonomic investigation and it is not yet possible to interpret them in neurological terms.

Contingent negative variation (CNV)

Relatively few systematic studies have been carried out on changes in the contingent negative variation during aging. This well-known late potential is recorded in normal subjects in the interval which precedes the execution of a pre-arranged motor response and which is initiated by a forewarning signal (Walter et al., 1964). The classical procedure is therefore made up of a succession of forewarning stimuli, S1, an interval of active waiting and the imperative stimulus, S2. Normally, the CNV has its maximum amplitude in frontal and central regions. It is more dependent on what the subject has to do than on the physical characteristics of the stimuli. Differences between the elderly and controls have been noticed in experiments on the effects at different interstimulus intervals. With intervals of several seconds, i.e. relatively long periods to wait for S2, the older subjects were found to develop smaller and more irregular CNVs than young controls (Loveless and Sanford, 1974). The findings are not consistent, however. Others have observed an increase in negativity before S2 in the aged even with a long interval (Schaie and Syndulko, 1977).

When subjects initiate the S1–S2 sequence themselves, the CNV is slightly smaller in amplitude in the elderly (Michalewski et al., 1979) though it is possible that subjects develop a spontaneous negativity before the test, introducing a ceiling effect which prevents further increases. Variations of memory abilities and personality have more effect on CNV than chronological age (Nakamura et al., 1979).

In a study on three groups of subjects (young, 60s and over 70s) subjects undertook an attention task designed to evoke a CNV (Tecce et al., 1982). In all three groups there is a reduction in the late components of the CNV but in the first two groups there is a rebound effect on trials that do not demand attention (there are significant elevations in late CNV amplitude). In addition, the early component of the CNV diminishes in all the groups when an attention task is involved but this reduction is present in the oldest subjects, even without such a task. These data may be explained by the difficulty the elderly subjects have in dividing their attention. We shall return to the question of divided attention in Chapter 8.

* * * * * *

As we have seen, the electrical activity recorded from the scalp contains many signals related to mental processes, including perception, cognition, attention, arousal and expectancy. Because it is non-invasive, electrophysiology is certain to retain a central role in studies of human brain function. However, a great deal remains to be done to define the changes which take place during aging. Many areas are inadequately documented and conflicting reports surround the magnitude and even the direction of some of the effects. Interpretation of many of the findings awaits a better understanding of the neurological generators of the recorded signals and of their psychological specificity. Nevertheless it is already possible to reach a number of important conclusions:

1. There is a small but significant reduction (<1 Hz) with age in the frequency of the predominant rhythm of the waking EEG.
2. The topographic distribution of EEG frequencies is preserved in normal old age.
3. EEG abnormalities are common in the normal elderly. However they are not peculiar to old age; their incidence increases progressively throughout life.
4. Some components of evoked potentials are delayed in old age. The late components associated with cognitive processes are more affected than the early components which reflect sensory processes.
5. Evoked response phenomena are highly sensitive to stimulus conditions and to demands placed upon the subject. Small changes in these variables can be sufficient to abolish age dependent effects.
6. Careful considerations must be given to the psychophysical condition of subjects who take part in electrophysiological studies of normal aging. The electrical activity of the brain is so sensitive to psychological variables such as mood and arousal, preoccupation with ailments and other problems, that it is easy for aging to become confounded with other variables.
7. Features of the power spectrum of the EEG and certain components of evoked potentials undergo marked changes in dementia. These effects promise more accurate differential diagnosis between dementia and other disorders of old age than is currently possible with neurochemical or brain imaging techniques.

REFERENCES

Abe, K., and Suzuki, T. (1985). Age trends of early awakening and feeling worse in the morning than in the evening in apparently normal people. *J. Nerv. Ment. Dis.* 173, 495–498.
Allison, T., Hume, A. L., Wood, C. C., and Goff, W. R. (1984). Development and aging changes in somatosensory, auditory and visual evoked potentials. *Electroenceph. Clin. Neurophysiol.*, 58, 14–24.
Angeleri, F., Provinciali, L., Signorino, M., Piana, C., and Salvolini, U. (1983). Ageing mind, depression and dementia: a neuropsychological, electrophysiological and CT approach to the clinical diagnosis. In A. Cecchini, G. Nappi and A. Arrigo (Eds), *Cerebral Pathology in Old Age*. Pavia: Emiras, pp. 91–102.
Beck, E. C., Swanson, C., and Dustman, R. E. (1980). Long latency components of the visually evoked potential in man: effects of aging. *Exp. Aging Res.*, 6, 523–545.
Bixler, O. E., Kales, A., Cadieux, R. J., Vela-Bueno, A., Jacoby, J. A., and Soldatos, C. R. (1985). Sleep apneic activity in older healthy subjects. *J. Appl. Physiol.*, 58, 1597–1601.

Boening, J. (1980). Evozierte Potentiale als neuropsychobiologische Korrelationsmatrix zentralnervoeser Alternvorgange. *Akt. Gerontol.*, 10, 557–568.
Brown, W. S., Marsh, J. T., and LaRue, A. (1982). Event-related potentials in psychiatry: differentiating depression and dementia in the elderly. *Bull. Los Angeles Neurol. Soc.*, 47, 91–107.
Brown, W. S., Marsh, J. T., and LaRue, A. (1983). Exponential electrophysiological aging: P3 latency. *Electroenceph. Clin. Neurophysiol.*, 55, 277–285.
Buchtal, F., and Rosenfalck, A. (1966). Evoked action potentials and conduction velocity in human sensory nerve. *Brain Res.*, 3, 1–122.
Busse, E. W. (1983). Electroencephalography. In B. Reisberg (Ed.), *Alzheimer's Disease: The Standard Reference.* New York: The Free Press, pp. 231–237.
Celesia, G. G., and Daly, R. F. (1977). Effects of aging on visual evoked responses. *Arch. Neurol.*, 34, 403–407.
Coben, L. A., Danzinger, W. L., and Berg, L. (1983). Frequency analysis of the resting awake EEG in mild senile dementia of Alzheimer type. *Electroenceph. Clin. Neurophysiol.*, 55, 372–380.
Dement, W. C., Laughton, E. M., and Carskadon, M. A. (1982). White paper on sleep and aging. *J. Amer. Geriatr. Soc.*, 30, 25–50.
Desmedt, J., and Cheron, G. (1980). Somatosensory evoked potentials to finger stimulation in healthy octogenarians and in young adults: wave form scalp topography and transit times of parietal and frontal components. *Electroenceph. Clin. Neurophysiol.*, 50, 404–425.
Dorfman, L. J., and Bosley, T. M. (1979). Age-related changes in peripheral and central nerve conduction in man. *Neurology*, 29, 38–44.
Duffy, F. H., Albert, M. S., McAnulty, G., and Garvey, A. J. (1984a). Age-related differences in brain electrical activity of healthy subjects. *Ann. Neurol.*, 16, 430–438.
Duffy, F. H., Albert, M. S., McAnulty, G., and Garvey, A. J. (1984b). Brain electrical activity in patients with presenile and senile dementia of the Alzheimer type. *Ann. Neurol.*, 16, 439–448.
Dustman, R. E., Snyder, R. W., and Schlehuber, C. J. (1981). Life-span alterations in visually evoked potentials and inhibitory functions. *Neurobiol. Aging*, 2, 187–192.
Fein, G., Feinburg, I., Insel, T. R., Antrobus, J. S., Price, L. J., Floyd, T. C., and Nelson, M. A. (1985). Sleep mentation in the elderly. *Psychophysiology*, 22, 218–225.
Ford, J. M., Hink, R. F., Hopkins, W. F., Roth, W. T., Pfefferbaum, A., and Kopell, B. S. (1979). Age effects on event-related potentials in a selective attention task. *J. Gerontol.*, 34, 388–395.
Gasser, T., Bacher, P., and Steinberg, H. (1985). Test–retest reliability of spectral parameters of the EEG. *Electroenceph. Clin. Neurophysiol.*, 60, 312–319.
Gastaut, H. (1974). Vom Berger-Rhythmus zum Alpha-Kult und zur Alpha-Kultur. EEG-EMG, 5, 189–199.
Gastaut, J. L., Farnarier, G., Michel, B., Serbanescu, T., Barrat, E., and Sambuc, R. (1980). Etude correlative des données EEG et scanographyques au cours du vieillissement cerebral normal et pathologique. *Rev. EEG Neurophysiol.*, 10, 228–235.
Gerson, I. M., and Chat, E. (1967). Electroencephalographic studies on the aging process: psychometric correlates. *J. Amer. Geriatr. Soc.*, 15, 185–190.
Gerson, I. M., John, R. E., Bartlett, F., and Koenig, V. (1976). Average evoked response (AER) in the electroencephalographic diagnosis of the normally aging brain. A practical application. *Clin. EEG*, 7, 77–91.
Giaquinto, S. (1980). Computerized EEG in the study of cerebral alteration and brain pathology in the aged. In G. Barbagallo-Sangiorgi and A. N. Exton-Smith (Eds), *The Aging Brain.* New York: Plenum Press, 229–239.
Giaquinto, S., and Nolfe, G. (1986). The EEG in the normal elderly: a contribution to the interpretation of aging and dementia. *Electroenceph. Clin. Neurophysiol.*, 63, 540–546.

Gordon, E. B., and Sim, M. (1967). The EEG in presenile dementia. *J. Neurol. Neurosurg. Psychiat.*, 30, 285–291.

Guggenheim, P., and Karbowski, K. (1979). EEG-Befunde bei 40–60 jahrigen gesunden. Probanden. *Z. Gerontol.*, 12, 365–375.

Harbin, T. J., Marsh, G. R., and Harvey, M. T. (1984). Differences in the late components of the event-related potential due to age and to semantic and non-semantic tasks. *Electroenceph. Clin. Neurophysiol.*, 59, 489–496.

Harding, G. F. A., Wright, C. E., and Orwin, A. (1985). Primary presenile dementia: the use of the visual evoked potential as a diagnostic indicator. *Brit. J. Psychiat.*, 147, 532–539.

Harner, R. N. (1975). EEG evaluation of the patient with dementia. In D. F. Benson and D. Blumer (Eds), *Psychiatric Aspects of Neurological Diseases*. New York: Grune & Stratton, pp. 63–82.

Hubbard, O., Sunde, D., and Goldensohn, E. S. (1976). The EEG in centenarians. *Electroenceph. Clin. Neurophysiol.*, 40: 407–417.

Hughes, J. R., and Cayaffa, J. J. (1977). The EEG in patients at different ages without organic cerebral disease. *Electroenceph. Clin. Neurophysiol.*, 42, 776–784.

Hume, A. L., Cant, B. R., Shaw, N. A., and Cowan, J. C. (1982). Central somatosensory conduction time from 10 to 79 years. *Electroenceph. Clin. Neurophysiol.*, 54, 49–54.

Jerger, J., and Hall, J. (1980). Effects of age and sex on auditory brain stem response. *Arch. Otolaryngol.*, 106, 387–395.

John, R. E., Karmel, B. Z., Corning, W. C., Easton, P., Brown, D., Ahn, H., John, M., Harmony, T., Princhep, L., Toro, A., Gerson, I., Bartless, F., Thatcher, R., Kaye, H., Valdes, P., and Schartz, E. E. (1977). Neurometrics. *Science*, 210, 1255–1258.

Kaszniak, A. W., Garron, D. C., Fox, J. H., Bergen, D., and Huckman, M. (1979). Cerebral atrophy, EEG slowing age, education and cognitive functioning in suspected dementia. *Neurology*, 29, 1273–1279.

Katz, R. I., and Horowitz, G. R. (1982). Electroencephalogram in the septuagenarians: studies in a normal geriatric population. *J. Amer. Geriatr. Soc.*, 3, 273–275.

Kazis, A., Karlovasitou, A., and Xafenias, D. (1982). Temporal slow activities of the EEG in old age. *Arch. Psychiat. Nervenkr.*, 231, 547–554.

Kooi, K. A., Guevener, A. M., Tupper, C. J., and Bagchi, B. K. (1964). Electroencephalographic patterns of the temperal regions in normal adults. *Neurology*, 14, 1029–1035.

Liston, E. H. (1979). Clinical findings in presenile dementia. *J. Nerv. Ment. Dis.*, 167,337–342.

Loveless, N. E., and Sanford, A. J. (1974). Effects of age on the contingent negative and preparatory set in a reaction-time task. *J. Gerontol.*, 29, 52–63.

Marsh, G. R., and Thompson, L. W. (1972). Age differences in evoked potentials during an auditory discrimination task. *Gerontologist*, 12, 44.

Matejcek, M. (1980). Application de l'analyse spectrale pour l'étude de certaines relations entre l'activitè EEG occipitale et l'age. *Rev. EEG Neurophysiol.*, 10, 122–130.

Matousek, M., Volavka, J., Roubicek, J., and Roth, Z. (1967). EEG frequency analysis related to age in normal adults. *Electroenceph. Clin. Neurophysiol.*, 23, 162–167.

Michalewski, H. T., Thompson, L. W., and Patterson, J. V. (1979). The role of EEG techniques in the assessment of life-span changes and responses to drugs. In A. Raskin and L. F. Jarvik (Eds), *Psychiatric Symptoms and Cognitive Loss in the Elderly*. New York: John Wiley & Sons, pp. 73–124.

Mullis, R. J., Holcomb, P. J., Diner, B. C., and Dykman, R. A. (1985). The effects of aging on the P3 component of the visual event-related potential. *Electroenceph. Clin. Neurophysiol.*, 62, 141–149.

Mundy-Castle, A., Hurst, L. A., Beerstecher, D., and Prinsloo, T. (1954). The electroencephalogram in the senile psychoses. *Electroenceph. Clin. Neurophysiol.*, 6, 245–252.

Nakamura, M., Fukui, Y., Kadobayashi, I., and Kato, N. (1979). A comparison of the

CNV in young and old subjects: its relation to memory and personality. *Electroenceph. Clin. Neurophysiol.*, 46, 337–344.

Neshige, R., Barrett, G., and Shibasaki, H. (1985). The change of P300 latency with age and its applications in the study of dementias. *J. Neurol.*, 232 (suppl.), 255.

Obrist, W. D., Sokoloff, L., Lassen, N. A., Lane, M. H., Butler, R. N., and Feinberg, I. (1963). Relation of EEG to cerebral blood flow and metabolism in old age. *Electroenceph. Clin. Neurophysiol.*, 15, 610–619.

Okudaira, N., Fukuda, H., Nishihara, K., Ohtani, K., Endo, S., and Torii, S. (1983). Sleep apnea and nocturnal myoclonus in elderly persons in Vilcabamba, Ecuador. *J. Gerontol.*, 38, 436–438.

Ono, K., Mameda, G., Shimada, D., and Yamashita, M. (1982). EEG correlation with intelligence test performance in senescence: a new pattern discriminative approach. *Int. J. Neurosci.*, 16, 47–52.

Otomo, E. (1966). Electroencephalography in old age: dominant alpha pattern. *Electroenceph. Clin. Neurophysiol.*, 21, 489–491.

Ott, H., McDonald, R. J., Fichte, K., and Herrmann, W. M. (1982). Interpretation of correlation between EEG-power-spectra and psychological performance variables within the concepts of subvigilance, attention and psychomotoric impulsion. In W. M. Herrmann (Ed.), *Electroencephalography in Drug Research*. Stuttgart: Fischer, pp. 227–247.

Patterson, M. B., Gluck, H., and Mack, J. L. (1983). EEG activity in the 13–15 Hz band correlates with intelligence in healthy elderly women. *Int. J. Neurosci.* 20, 161–172.

Penttila, M., Partanen, J. V., Soininen, H., and Riekkinen, P. J. (1985). Quantitative analysis of occipital EEG in different stages of Alzheimer's disease. *Electroenceph. Clin. Neurophysiol.*, 60, 1–6.

Pfefferbaum, A., Ford, J. M., Roth, W. T., Hopkins, W. F., and Kopell, B. S. (1979). Event-related potential changes in healthy aged females. *Electroenceph. Clin. Neurophysiol.*, 46, 81–86.

Pfefferbaum, A., Ford, J. M., Roth, W. T., and Kopell, B. S. (1980a). Age differences in P3-reaction time associations. *Electroenceph. Clin. Neurophysiol.*, 49, 257–265.

Pfefferbaum, A., Ford, J. M., Roth, W. T., and Kopell, B. S. (1980b). Age-related changes in auditory event-related potentials. *Electroenceph. Clin. Neurophysiol.*, 49, 266–276.

Pfefferbaum, A., Ford, J. M., Wenegrat, B. G., Roth, W. T., and Kopell, B. S. (1984). Clinical application of the P3 component of event-related potentials. *Electroenceph. Clin. Neurophysiol.*, 59, 85–103.

Podlesny, J. A., and Dustman, R. E. (1982). Age effects on heart rate, sustained potential and P3 responses during reaction-time tasks. *Neurobiol. Aging*, 3, 1–9.

Podlesny, J. A., Dustman, R. E., and Shearer, D. E. (1984). Aging and respond–withhold tasks: effects on sustained potentials, P3 responses and late activity. *Electroenceph. Clin. Neurophysiol.*, 58, 130–139.

Polich, J., Howard, L., and Starr, A. (1985). Effects of age on the P300 component of the event-related potential from auditory stimuli: peak definition, variation, and measurement. *J. Gerontol.*, 40, 721–726.

Prinz, P. N., Peskind, E. R., Vitaliano, P. P., Raskind, M. A., Eisdorfer, C., Zemcuznikov, N., and Gerber, C. V. (1982). Changes in the sleep and waking EEGs of nondemented and demented elderly subjects. *J. Amer. Geriat. Soc.*, 30, 86–93.

Reynolds III, C. F., Kupfer, D. J., Taska, L. S., Hoch, C. C., Sewitch, D. E., and Spiker, D. G. (1985). Sleep of healthy seniors: a revisit. *Sleep*, 8, 20–29.

Roberts, M. A., McGeorge, A. P., and Caird, F. I. (1978). Electroencephalography and computerized tomography in vascular and non-vascular dementia in old age. *J. Neurol. Neurosurg. Psychiat.*, 41, 903–906.

Rossini, P. M., Onofrj, M., Gambi, D., Sollazzo, D., and Lomonaco, M. (1979). Il potenziale evocato acustico troncoencefalico (BSEP) in soggetti normali a diverse età. *Riv. Ital. EEG Neurofisiol. Clin.*, 2, 587–589.

Roubicek, J. (1977). The electroencephalogram in the middle-aged and the elderly. *J. Amer. Geriatr. Soc.,* 25, 145–152.

Rowe, M. J. (1978). Normal variability of the brain stem auditory evoked response in young and old adult subjects. *Electroenceph. Clin. Neurophysiol.,* 44, 459–470.

Schaie, J. P., and Syndulko, K. (1977). CNV components and cardiac correlates of time estimation and reaction time performance in the elderly. *Psychophysiology,* 14, 92.

Silverman, A. J., Busse, E. W., and Barnes, R. H. (1955). Studies in the process of aging: electroencephalographic findings in 400 elderly subjects. *Electroenceph. Clin. Neurophysiol.,* 7, 67–74.

Simpson, D. M., and Erwin, C. W. (1983). Evoked potential latency change with age suggests differential aging of primary somatosensory cortex. *Neurobiol. of Aging,* 4, 59–63.

Smith, J. R., Karacan, I., and Yang, M. (1977). Ontogeny of delta activity during human sleep. *Electroenceph. Clin. Neurophysiol.,* 43, 229–237.

Snyder, E. W., Dustman, R. E., and Shearer, D. E. (1981). Pattern reversal evoked potential amplitude: life span changes. *Electroenceph. Clin. Neurophysiol.,* 52, 429–434.

Soininen, H., Partanen, V. J., Helkala, E. L., and Riekkinen, P. J. (1982). EEG findings in senile dementia and normal aging. *Acta Neurol. Scand.,* 65, 59–70.

Sokoloff, L. (1966). Cerebral circulatory and metabolic changes associated with aging. *Res. Publ. Ass. Nerv. Ment. Dis.,* 41, 237–254.

Stefoski, D., Bergen, D., Fox, J., Morrell, F., Huckman, M. and Ramsey, R. (1976). Correlation between diffuse EEG abnormalities and cerebral atrophy in senile dementia. *J. Neurol. Neurosurg. Psychiat.,* 39, 751–755.

Straumanis, J. J., Shagass, C., and Schwartz, M. (1965). Visually evoked cerebral response changes associated with chronic brain syndrome and aging. *J. Gerontol.,* 20, 498–506.

Tecce, J. J., Cattanach, L., Yrchik, D. A., and Meinbresse, D. (1982). CNV rebound and aging. *Electroenceph. Clin. Neurophysiol.,* 54, 175–186.

Torres, F., Faoro, A., Loewenson, R., and Johnson, E. (1983). The electroencephalogram of elderly subjects revisited. *Electroenceph. Clin. Neurophysiol.,* 56, 391–398.

Trojaborg, W. (1976). Motor and sensory conduction in the musculocutaneous nerve. *J. Neurol. Neurosurg. Psychiat.,* 39, 890–899.

Visser, S. L., Van Tilburg, W., Hooijer, C., Jonker, C., and De Rijke, W. (1985). Visual evoked potentials (VEPs) in senile dementia (Alzheimer type) and in non-organic behavioural disorders in the elderly: comparison with EEG parameters. *Electroenceph. Clin. Neurophysiol.,* 60, 115–121.

Walter, W. G., Cooper, R., Aldridge, V. J., McCallum, W. C., and Winter, A. L. (1964). Contingent negative variations: an electric sign of sensorimotor association and expectancy in the human brain. *Nature,* 203, 380–384.

Wang, H. S., and Busse, E. W. (1969). EEG of healthy old persons — A longitudinal study. I. Dominant background activity and occipital rhythm. *J. Gerontol.,* 24, 419–426.

Wang, H. S., Obrist, W. D., and Busse, E. W. (1974). Neurophysiological correlates of the intellectual function. In E. Palmore (Ed.), *Normal Aging II.* Durham, N. C.: The Duke University Press, pp. 115–126.

Webb, W. B. (1985). A further analysis of age and sleep deprivation effects. *Psychophysiology,* 22, 156–161.

Wright, C. E., Harding, G. F. A., and Orwin, A. (1984). Pre-senile dementia—the use of the flash and pattern VEP in diagnosis. *Electroenceph. Clin. Neurophysiol.,* 57, 405–415.

Wright, C. E., Williams, D. E., Drasdo, N., and Harding, G. F. A. (1985). The influence of age on the electroretinogram and visual evoked potential. *Doc. Opthalmol.,* 59, 365–384.

Wright, E. A., and Gilmore, R. L. (1985). Features of geriatric EEG: age-dependent incidence of POSTS. *Clin. Electroencephalogr.,* 16, 11–15.

CHAPTER 8

Cognitive activity and personality

The speed of processing in the aging nervous system undergoes changes which parallel the age-dependent variations in electrophysiological markers. Both are different from the changes which occur in true dementia. The altered timing does not affect familiar activities in everyday life.

The published work on cerebral aging is copious, meticulous and growing. No area of aging research is broader than that of neuropsychology and in this field a longstanding dispute exists over the effects of aging on cognitive abilities. The early literature is clouded by the contradictory findings of poorly controlled and even deliberately biased experiments. More recently neuropsychologists have acknowledged the importance of rigorously designed experiments and a large body of evidence has begun to accumulate. It is our personal belief that the neuropsychological data on aging should not be considered in isolation but integrated with other measures of cerebral function provided by neurochemistry and neurophysiology.

First of all, any study of age-dependent variation in higher nervous activity must distinguish between changes in cognitive activity itself and those which are secondary to deterioration in peripheral sensory mechanisms. As St Thomas (1225–1274) pointed out, '*nihil est in intellectu quod prius non fuerit in sensu*', nothing is in the mind that did not first come through the senses. We shall see how extensively the peripheral sensory pathways are affected by aging in the next chapter. For the time being it is sufficient to realize the potential for misinterpretation if these factors are not taken into account. Consider, for example, how cognitive activity may be held up and its effectiveness impaired by the purely sensory disorders of hearing and sight which are so common in old age. Such factors must therefore be carefully controlled in any neuropsychological investigation of aging.

Of course it is not possible to separate the processes of sensation, perception and cognition entirely. Subjectively, they are part of a mental continuum. Experimental psychology has demonstrated so many interactions between what were once considered successive stages in information processing that their boundaries have all but vanished. Nevertheless we shall fall back on these simple concepts in the sections which follow, for the sake of clarity.

ATTENTION

Attention has been defined in many different ways. One which is useful in the framework of the present discussion describes it as 'the capacity or energy to support cognitive processing' (Plude and Hoyer, 1985). Attention is not seen as a unitary process, because it can be referred to a specific sensory input (for example, visual attention) or to a specific strategy (for example, effortful versus automatic attention) or to a task-related goal (for example, memory organization and retrieval). In Plude and Hoyer's model, attention has been considered as a filter, that prevents the over-load in a system with limited capacity. It is still under discussion whether there are separate resources for each attention channel or a single function of capacity and energy shared by all. Preattentive processes have also been identified. They operate without placing demands on the limited capacity of the system, without awareness and without directed control. They are different from automatic attention, a process that consumes little energy and is based on overlearned sequences. Automatic encoding draws little upon the limited capacity of the central processing. On the other hand, effortful encoding places a strain on the processing capacity.

There are data supporting the view that the processes of automatic attention do not change with age. Although automatic attention can be acquired by overlearning functions that were once (like riding a bicycle) effortful, it is argued that some processes are inherently automatic; humans are genetically prepared for them and these processes do not alter in old age (Hasher and Zacks, 1979). This important study regards effortful and automatic processing as the opposite ends of a continuum. Effortful processing diminishes the ability to deal with other effortful activities. Automatic processing is not improved by practice and does not require awareness.

Effortful attention can be either focused or divided. Focused attention is not affected by aging. For example, in an experiment in which subjects had to sort cards according to the presence of a T at a particular location on the card, the presence of dissimilar nontargets did not slow the performance of elderly subjects (Farkas and Hoyer, 1980). However, the same study found that elderly adults were slowed by dissimilar targets when the targets might be located in any one of four positions on the card, thus calling for a visual search and divided attention. A low complexity in the visual search for letters improves the performance in the elderly subjects, since it is supposed that targets will be detected with the help of automatic attention. Older adults may benefit even more than younger adults when uncertainty about the spatial location of target information is reduced (Madden and Nebes, 1980; Madden, 1984). Nissen and Corkin (1985) demonstrated that spatial and temporal expectancy was useful for both elderly and younger controls. In their experiments a visual warning cue was represented by an arrow pointing either right or left. In 80% of their presentations the target letter was displayed on the side indicated by the arrow. In a third of cases a double arrow meant that the right and left locations were equally likely. Responses of both groups were also faster on trials with a 3 sec warning interval compared to a 2 sec warning interval. In conclusion, the former view of an age-dependent decrease in the ability to ignore irrelevant stimuli has been modified by stating that the decrease is not seen when 'neutral noise' borders the target situation in a non-search task (Wright and Elias, 1979). In these experiments the perceptual intrusions were equivalent in both elderly subjects and young controls.

Divided attention is called for when different but relevant stimuli are presented at the same time (for example, in a condition consisting of a primary mental reasoning task and a concurrent memory task). Automatic attention acquired by over-learning is said to be helpful, because one or more of the information processing systems demands less energy, thus permitting a lesser load on cognitive abilities and consequently better performance in time-demanding tasks. On the other hand, when tasks or everyday life involve at least two competing sources of information, attention must usually be switched between them so that the processing of one channel decreases the ability to process the other. It has been shown that the ability to process more than one channel of information declines with age, whether performance is expressed in terms of response time or accuracy, suggesting a decreased capacity of attentional system. In our laboratory a system used for investigating divided attention shows that young controls outscore elderly subjects only on the hardest tasks (Fig. 8.1). The reaction time for detecting a target letter is longer if it is presented among nontargets in the display than it is presented alone. Reaction time increases by 50% in older subjects and by 37% for younger controls, when the target may appear at any one of several positions on the screen. On the other hand, in a non-search task, that is to say when the target appears only in the centre position of the display, the perceptual intrusions increase reaction time by only 8% for elderly subjects with equivalent age-related attentional selectivity, which is a process which allocate mental resources of limited capacity among concomitant stimuli (see Plude and Hoyer, 1985). In the previous chapter we saw neurophysiological evidence for differences in the way the elderly cope with divided loads on their attention. The CNV varied in young subjects according to the attentional demands of each trial. In subjects over 70 the late phase of CNV did not alter with changing stimulus conditions. The interference impairs the possibility of dividing attention either by filling the general capacity or limiting the activity in focal structure-specific channels.

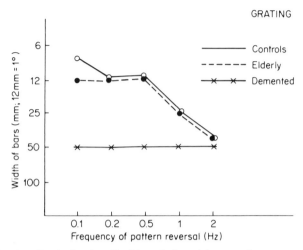

Fig. 8.1   Grating discrimination. In this task the subject watches a screen and has to count the number of 'moving' white bars in the upper half field. Each point indicates the width threshold for each frequency. Elderly subjects differ from young controls in the finest visual resolution. The groups overlap only when large bars are used

REACTION TIME

Reaction time can be measured in a wide variety of conditions, and it can be used to test both focused and divided attention. Although it has been widely used in experimental psychology a number of authors have recently drawn attention to the methodological difficulties (e.g. McCormack, 1984; Salthouse, 1985). There is nevertheless general agreement that reaction time slows with age, and that the effect is beyond the volitional control of the individual. There is an alternative view that older subjects are deliberately slower because they are concerned with accuracy, thus suggesting that they prefer to trade speed for accuracy. In our experiments on the detection of visually presented letters, the number of errors does not vary significantly with age; on the other hand the number of omissions increases, indicating a 'conservative' attitude (Table 8.1). However, we calculate

Table 8.1   Choice reaction time. Hit probability (HP) and omission probability (OP)

Probability	Elderly	Controls
HP	0.943	0.982
OP	0.057	0.018 P < .05

that between the ages of 20 and 60, a decline of 5–15% occurs in speed of response. This would appear to argue against any simple trade off of speed for accuracy. From a methodological point of view, Salthouse has proposed that the speed–accuracy tradeoff should be determined within individuals in order to make appropriate corrections for incorrect responses in calculating average reaction time (Salthouse, 1985). It is important to remember that all elderly people are not equally affected by slowing. In a study of people aged 58–75 (mean age 64.8) Smith and Brewer (1985) found some elderly subjects as fast as younger controls. As we saw in the case of evoked potentials, a number of physiological and psychological variables affect the magnitude of any slowing in reaction time. The effect may be minimal if subjects are adequately prepared for the task and when peripheral factors, such as hearing loss, are controlled for (Gottsdanker, 1982). As in other trained tasks (Chapter 12), factors such as warning signals, practice, positive verbal reinforcement and monetary reward all improve performance. It also appears that age related increments in reaction time are not present when subjects respond vocally rather than manually, suggesting that vocal programming is more resistant to the effects of aging (Nebes, 1978).

Slowing of reaction time with age cannot be accounted for entirely by changes in peripheral pathways. The manipulation of the quality of external stimuli affects only the encoding stage of processing which is indicated as a primary locus of slowing in information processing with age (Simon and Pouraghabagher, 1978). By simulating the neural network Salthouse (1985) showed that the consequences of processing rate are within certain limits independent of peripheral factors like the duration of external stimulation and the transmission time. Obviously, central processing efficiency depends on peripheral factors, but it is unlikely that peripheral variations have widespead effects throughout the system. The simple computer simulation employed by Salthouse shows more pronounced effects when the 'rate' variable is active at a higher level of the network.

In our experiments there was no slowing in colour recognition in elderly subjects (Table 8.2). Subtracting simple reaction time (no discrimination) from

Table 8.2   Tachistoscopy for colours (msec)

Group	Red	Yellow	Blue	Significance
Controls	18	18	18	
Elderly	18	18	18	
Demented	157	2525	1782	P < .0001
		Accuracy		
Controls	100%	100%	100%	
Elderly	100%	100%	100%	
Demented	64%	64%	43%	P < .0001

choice reaction time in the same subjects removes variables due to peripheral conduction time and reveals that central processes are slowed in the elderly (Fig. 8.2). The difference between choice reaction time (colour discrimination) and

REACTION TIMES

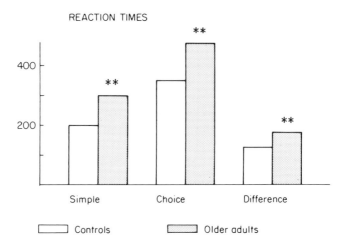

Fig. 8.2 Simple and choice reaction times in elderly subjects and young controls. Times are longer with increasing age. The subtractive method shows a greater difference in the elderly, thus indicating a central locus of slowing

simple reaction time (no discrimination) is 71 msec in the elderly, a value similar to that (75 msec) found in experiments on relatedness (name identity vs. physical identity) in paired stimulus letters (Hines and Posner, quoted by Kausler, 1982). In trials on letter identification with backward masking there is a 30 msec difference between elderly and younger subjects (Walsh et al., 1979) The slowed operation is not offset by the stimulus persistence. The 30 msec delay is less than the 71–75 msec in our own observations and those for Hines and Posner because discrimination and motor decision are not involved.

Changes in central processing time are probably reflected in the electrophysiological data. If 'the time between the second wave of the visual evoked response and the linked premotor potential' is measured, the interval is found to increase in a linear fashion with age at the rate of 1.4 msec/yr (Smith et al., 1985). The changes are probably also reflected in the increased latency of late waves of the evoked response described in the last chapter, in particular of N2.

There is an extensive literature on differences in the number of errors between elderly subjects and younger controls. A 'conservative' attitude is gained with age. The elderly score fewer hits for true signals embedded in noise than do the 'liberal' young, but they make fewer false positive responses than younger subjects (Kausler, 1982). A response bias is therefore brought about by age, but it does not necessarily mean a change in mental ability.

Reaction time may be regarded as the sum of a number of different processes each with its own duration. An analysis identifies five factors in the control of motor response, named baseline factor, promotor factor, motor factor, force factor and release factor (Vrtunski et al, 1984). The last one is the most consistent in distinguishing young and elderly groups and is considered by the authors as the 'purest' measure of age changes. The premotor segment is the interval of cognitive activity including preprocessing, feature extraction, identification, decision making and response programming. A variable, called by these authors 'maximum speed', discriminates elderly subjects from controls, as does the variable called 'response duration', expressing the interval during which the force exceeds a certain level.

More demanding choice reaction time tasks lead to greater short-term exhaustion, but the effect of age on endurance is not evident up to age 65 (Gottsdanker, 1984). If subjects are given information about their speed and accuracy, this feedback speeds up the reaction time of the young resulting in a higher number of errors but it slows the responses of the elderly subjects (Hines, 1979).

INPUT PROCESSING

Reading letters from a display requires the extraction of information from a sensory buffer. This form of storage is called 'iconic' in the case of visual patterns and 'echoic' in the case of auditory ones. Cerella et al. (1982) have shown that there is an age-dependent slowing in the rate at which information is extracted from these buffers. Elderly subjects are slower by a factor of 1.31 (the iconic read-out is 27 msec/letter for the young and 35 msec/letter for the old). The age effect is more intense when multi-element displays are involved. Nevertheless, this simple extraction of information is relatively spared by age, in comparison with the processes involved in transformation and storage of information which are slowed by a factor of 1.7–1.8.

There is a significant decrease in extrafoveal perception of age. A moderate deficit in letter identification in the fovea is larger in the periphery. When the retinal eccentricity of a target is shifted from $0°$ to $2°$ its identification time is doubled in the elderly. Older subjects' performance is also impaired by near distractors (Cerella, 1985). In this experiment visual stimuli are delivered to the subject, consisting of a centred letter (the target) sandwiched by a pair of matched letters (the distractors). For example, the shift of small (2/16 in high letters) and incongruous (i.e. RGR) distractors to $\pm 0.7°$ takes 76 msec longer to identify in the elderly. If the same distractors are shifted to $\pm 1.4°$ the difference becomes 71 msec, whereas if they are shifted to $3.75°$ the difference is only 57 msec. Thus distracting stimuli exert a reduced effect of interference in the elderly when they are located outside the fovea.

The elderly subject is able to see only a limited number of patterns simultaneously. His search calls for more fixations, as if his perceptual window had shrunk. A deficit in perceptual organization is seen in other experiments. Both young and elderly subjects can take advantage of the chunking and grouping of similar visual information, which permits the isolation of a target in a small context. However, in the case of large perceptual units, the elderly are unable to engender the organization implied by the Gestalt principles of grouping by proximity or similarity in finding a target (Gilmore et al., 1985). The ability to identify incomplete pictures given partial visual information is also impaired in normal aging. In one study using the least complete set of images, a young group identified 67% of the pictures, whereas an old normal group and patients affected by Alzheimer's disease could identify only 31% and 16% respectively (Rissenberg, 1985).

In the elderly, stimulus images persist longer in the nervous system. If half of each letter of a series of three-letter words is presented to a subject followed by the remaining part after a variable interval, older adults identify more total words than the young (Kline and Orme-Rogers, 1978). This is one of the few examples where elderly subjects outscore younger controls. But, enhanced stimulus-persistence is relatively unfavourable, since successive information does not find available synaptic pathways to process it. The neural representation of the first stimulus needs to be 'cleared through the nervous system' before the second stimulus can be processed. Stimulus-persistence leaves the responder either relatively refractory to subsequent stimulation or, more often, 'responsive but in a different way' (Botwinick, 1978) Thus, the young can take advantage of the shorter stimulus persistence to process information from sensory buffers at a higher rate.

The stimulus-persistence effect is confirmed by experiments on critical flicker frequency fusion (CFF). When a light or a chequer-board pattern is flashed on and off at an increasing rate, the stimulus will eventually be seen as steadily on. The rate at which fusion first takes place is the CFF. CFF can also be determined by starting from steady-state conditions and increasing the dark interval until separated flashes of light or chequer-board patterns are seen. In a study in which the stimuli were flashes of light, the elderly perceived the fusion point at a slower rate of flickering than younger controls (Falk and Kline, 1978). The mean dark interval threshold was found to be greater than 90 msec for the elderly (owing to the greater persistence in this group) and only about 65 msec in young subjects (Amberson et al., 1979). In our observations, where incidentally we equate pupil size between subjects by the use of atropine, fusion has also been found to take place at a lower rate in the elderly (Fig. 8.3). However, all these measurements of CFF may be biased, because the elderly adopt a 'conservative' criterion of fusion emphasizing any difference from the young subjects. Although the CFF studies support the concept of extended stimulus persistence in the elderly, at least one finding seems to indicate an opposite effect. Other observations are contrary to the persistence concept. Visual storage was found to persist 15% longer in the young than in elderly subjects in experiments where a circle was alternated with a blank interval (Walsh and Thompson, 1978). A variety of factors may influence the results of such studies, however, including the luminance and contrast of the stimuli and the opportunity for practice to achieve stable judgements.

Increased stimulus persistence in the elderly can be accounted for by differential aging of the transient versus the sustained visual channels of the visual pathway (Kline, 1984). The former respond quickly and briefly to changes in visual stimulation, whereas the latter are slow to respond, produce long-lasting effects and integrate stimulus energy over long time intervals. According to Kline, there is a shift in the nervous system towards a sustained type of functioning, with a decreased detection of low-spatial frequencies and moving or flickering patterns. Clearly this may result from the loss of neurons in the optic tracts which we have discussed in early chapters and which might effect transient cells selectively.

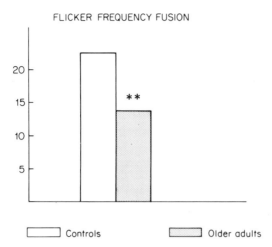

Fig. 8.3 Critical Flicker Fusion Frequency. Black and white chequer-board (6° × 8°), 100% contrast, 3 lux, 72 msec exposition. Mean values are obtained by increasing and decreasing the duration of the dark interval. The lower values in the elderly tally well with the hypothesis of a longer visual persistence. The values in patterns/sec correspond to 22.98/sec and 14.08/sec

BEHAVIOURAL SLOWING

According to a widely accepted theory, normal aging is associated with some form of slowing in the central nervous system which reduces the rate of cognitive processing and accounts for a variety of cognitive deficits that often come with old age (Birren, 1974; Salthouse and Somberg, 1982a and b). Cerebral functions are not all affected by this slowing down. Over-trained and inbuilt processes that take place automatically with very little load on cognitive systems appear to be largely untouched. For example, there appear to be no changes in size or brightness constancy with aging (Kausler, 1982). On the other hand cognitive processes seem particularly vulnerable as evidenced both by neuropsychological tests and changes in attendant electrophysiological events.

An explanation for the slowing of behaviour in terms of 'signal-to-noise ratio' has been offered by Welford (1985). The hypothesis suggests that the signal-to-noise ratio is degraded in the aging brain. As a result, the elderly take longer than the young to decide that a stimulus is present, to discriminate it and decide on a course of action. The mechanism is comparable with the necessity to slow speech on a noisy telephone or radio link in order to ensure reception of the message, except that in the case of the elderly the elevated 'noise' is endogenous, neural noise. It may be due to degenerative changes in either afferent pathways or central systems. In either case, normal safety margins will be lost so that the elderly also become more susceptible to exogenous noise in sensory channels. We shall examine degenerative changes in the afferent system in a subsequent chapter; we have already considered central changes in the elderly that may, for example, degrade signal processing in the case of visual contours and delay associated electrical activity.

This hypothesis has been tested in a number of ways in experiments designed to simulate aging (Salthouse and Lichty, 1985). Thus, reaction times lengthen in young subjects when background activity is increased or when the signal to respond is decreased in strength, or distorted. At levels of high simulated noise, the amount of stimulus distortion that can be tolerated is low. Conversely, with high levels of stimulus distortion, the amount of background noise that can be tolerated is low. However, when elderly and control subjects are tested, age differences are seen in reaction time itself, but not for either the noise or distortion thresholds, even if participants can take as long as they like. The authors conclude that the hypothesis of a decreased signal-to-noise ratio is only partly tenable.

There are two main types of psychological explanation for slowing of behaviour in old age, the 'determinant' and the 'consequence' positions. The former means that changes in the central nervous system determine speed of performance. Interference with mental abilities is secondary to this. Decline of performance is greater in difficult and paced tasks, when the demand increases to a point at which capacities are overloaded, or when efficient and novel use of control processes is required (e.g. Cunningham, 1980; Cerella et al., 1980; Burke and Light, 1981; Rabbitt, 1977; Plude and Hoyer, 1985; Welford, 1985). Birren et al. (1983) take the view that 'with regard to specific abilities, there seems to be rather good consensus that intellectual tasks involving a high speed component usually tend to show age decrease in most individuals fairly early; usually in the 30s. Ability tasks that are commonly utilized in everyday life tend to be insensitive to age'. Three somewhat different models fall within the 'determinant' framework (Table 8.3).

Table 8.3   Three models from the determinant perspective (Botwinick, 1984)

Additive model
$RT_0 = RT_y + c$
(as the task becomes difficult, the response time of the old and the young will slow to an equal extent: c is a CONSTANT)

Multiplicative model
$RT_0 = RT_y \times c$
(as the task becomes difficult, the response time of the old becomes relatively greater)

Exponential model
$RT_0 = RT_y^c$
(as the task becomes difficult, the slowing with age no longer increases linearly)

Speed of performance represents an important dimension in understanding the reasons for age-dependent differences. The time or rate of processing is assumed to be the critical factor at least for those cognitive activities that are minimally influenced by experience, as opposed to those which depend on cumulated knowledge and are presumed to either improve or remain stable with age (Salthouse, 1985). The 'universal decrement principle' argues that slowing in the central nervous system accounts for virtually all age-dependent changes in behavioural activities. This principle is challenged by many negative findings (Kausler, 1982), which we shall discuss later on. However, from the 'determinant' perspective it is admitted that 'the decision to concentrate only on measures thought to be relatively free of experiential influences is based on a desire to examine presumably basic aging processes, and not because of a belief that such measures provide the best or most valid means of assessing cognitive functioning and intellectual ability' (Salthouse, 1985).

The 'consequence' position holds that performance is slower with age because cognitive abilities decline. Speed of performance is not the only measure, since accuracy, problem solving or job performance are other kinds of evaluation.

Psychological discussion of the slowing of behaviour must be set against the biological data. It is very unlikely that changes in the central nervous system, such as the loss of neurons and alterations in the neurotransmitters, occur without parallel changes in the speed of processing. Consider, for example, the effect of changes in the dendritic arborization of nerve cells. Transfer of inhibitory post-synaptic potentials and excitatory post-synaptic potentials by electrotonic cable properties of the dendritic tree are integrated on the cell soma to determine whether or not an action potential is elicited at the axon hillock. The size of the dendritic field depends on the number and length of the dendrites and the density of synaptic spines which end on them. It is also conceivable that changes in dendritic arborization during aging impair the electrotonic conduction from dendrites of one cell to those of another, a mechanism providing fast interaction between cells (Schmitt et al., 1976). Such events might explain central slowing, at least in part. A schematic representation is displayed in Fig. 8.4.

Small changes in levels of neurotransmitters which do not lead to actual mental decay may nevertheless slow neural transmission. This could happen if, for example, there were a lowered rate of rate limiting enzyme actions, such as the hydroxylation of tyrosine to DOPA, or of choline uptake. Cognitive abilities that call for either dopaminergic or cholinergic transmission could be affected, when the demand upon these systems is high.

MEMORY

Loss of memory is a common complaint among the elderly and even among middle-aged people. As we shall see in Chapter 10, some memory deficits are 'benign' and it is perfectly normal for young people to forget much that they should have learned at school. These are not causes for concern. On the other hand, lapses of memory in the elderly raise the spectre of dementia. Elderly people certainly have poorer memories. Their complaints are usually about episodic memory, the ability to recall personal experiences. Data accumulated from the literature on performance on Wechsler Memory Scale reveal that visual reproduction shows the steepest drop with age. Cohorts closest to one another in age show significantly different performances, but there are cases where the older

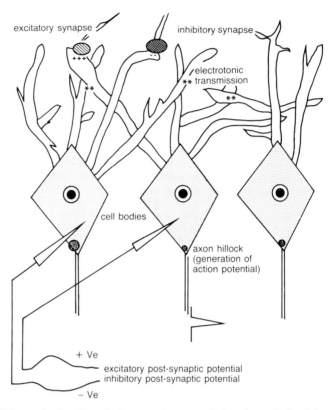

excitatory synapse

inhibitory synapse

electrotonic
transmission

cell bodies

axon hillock
(generation of
action potential)

+ Ve

excitatory post-synaptic potential
inhibitory post-synaptic potential

– Ve

Fig. 8.4 Schematic drawing of electrotonic transmission through dendrites. Their reduction with age might result in a slower and reduced throughput of information

group does not perform less efficiently (Margolis and Scialfa, 1984). Difficulty with visual memory has an important bearing on everyday activities, like face recognition (Ferris et al., 1980), a deficit that casts doubt on the reliability of elderly subjects as witnesses.

We have already considered age changes in sensory memory, the iconic and the echoic buffers. In the sections which follow we shall see the locus of central memory loss by considering encoding, storage and retrieval as separate processes.

Encoding

Encoding may be regarded as the first stage of learning, in which the information to be remembered is perceived and selected. Experimental studies on memory reveal that elderly people, as in other respects, are not a uniform group. For example, monetary reward, especially for the correct responses, improves learning because it is thought to favour the conditions for encoding, but it is effective only among elderly subjects from low socio-economic groups. Instructions on how to organize information from long lists of words also favours encoding but it helps only those elderly subjects of low verbal ability. Subjects of high verbal ability learn word lists with equal facility irrespective of age (see Botwinick, 1984). Similarly, under intentional learning (i.e. when a cognitive process is purposefully elaborated), there is an age deficit for the recognition of short segments of TV programs but only in those elderly subjects of low verbal ability (Cavanaugh, 1983). Practice through long experience may have a bearing on memory performance. For example, waiters who are used to remembering the orders of many customers perform well when tested for their recall of verbal material. The assessment of memory changes is subject to cohort effects unrelated to aging itself. Young people are used to the presence of an examiner, organizing their material, selecting efficient strategies, and to taking advantage of new educational methods. They are more able to work under conditions that require divided attention. They are less anxious, and more involved in learning and in challenging games in everyday life. Young people are continuously stimulated as well, whereas elderly people may be confused by laboratory tests, like paired associate learning, with which they are unfamiliar. Some authorities are inclined to play down the importance of cohort effects on the grounds that young adults of different generations have obtained similar scores in laboratory tests, while the cohort effect would be expected to favour the most recent generation. For this reason it is argued that laboratory measures provide a valid index of age-dependent changes (Kausler, 1982 and 1985). Cohort effects are largely avoided in longitudinal studies. We shall consider data of this type later in this chapter.

Encoding is also influenced by the kind of information to be processed. Meaningful words for successive transmission to long-term stores are processed automatically, apparently without effort, being innately programmed (Hasher and Zacks, 1979). This automatic conduction is independent of age. There is a large body of evidence that meaningless and unrelated material is poorly learned by the elderly. In a lexical task, where the old person has to tell whether a string of letters forms a word, latency and accuracy are unaffected by age (Bowles and Poon, 1985). On the other hand meaningless sentences presented at high speed are relatively poorly perceived, since elderly subjects are penalized by time compression (425 words per minute, more than twice the rate of normal conversation), but recall is excellent even at that rate when normal five- and eight-word sentences are read to the subject (Wingfield et al., 1985). There is also evidence that elderly subjects can outscore young controls when the words to be remembered are familiar to that generation (Barrett and Wright, 1981). They perform equally well for elderly- and both-cohort meaningful conditions, but obviously the young adults recall more of the young-meaningful list items (Hanley-Dunn and McIntosh, 1984). Colour memory declines with age, but performance improves when coloured pictures or symbols are related to an environmentally familiar context in everyday activities (Park and Puglisi, 1985). In the same research, the elderly were found to recall pictures better than words but not more so than young people. Moreover, many memory problems of elderly subjects are internally rather than externally generated, like statements, devices from their own experience and knowledge. For example, a young subject could score 26 at first trial in a backward digit span test, by forming two-figure numbers, giving each of them its name in 'lotto', a popular Italian game (a sort of 'bingo'), and finally grouping these names in a significant story.

Depression and cognitive impairment are correlated and some intellectual tasks are more affected by mood than by age itself. Provision of precise elaborations produces better encoding and better retention of target words, with no age differences, because it permits the individual to encode more aspects of the sentence context (Rankin and Collins, 1985). Clear semantic relations between the times to be remembered and a familiar context improves this contextual information (Hess, 1985). Elderly adults can then improve memory performance by better use of their semantic knowledge. Since older subjects derive more help from context than younger adults, their semantic organization is not impaired and can be used to facilitate word recognition (Cohen and Faulkner, 1983).

An active auditory rule improves performance, in many cases even more than visual input (see Botwinick, 1984). Roman people often read aloud and the Latin word meaning 'to say' has the same root as the Italian word 'to read'. A psychophysiological explanation for the usefulness of this channel in information processing is the longer duration of the auditory store compared to the visual one (Watkins and Watkins, 1980).

Storage

While changes in encoding abilities are well demonstrated and are supposed to be either the main or the only locus of memory deficit with age, storage problems do not exist (Smith, 1980). A theory of forgetting holds that elderly subjects are particularly susceptible to interference. As measured by retroactive inhibition, there does not appear to be a pronounced adult age difference in the rate of forgetting when the age groups are taken to the same criterion of mastery. However, some methodological problems arise in this case, because elderly subjects need additional trials and part of the material to be remembered is overlearned (see Kausler, 1982).

Retrieval and recall

Recall involves the search and retrieval of information that was previously encoded and stored. Recognition memory has been considered to be retrieval-free and therefore without age-effects. This contention is at odds with several investigations, which indicate reliable age differences with a variety of materials such as words, pictures or photographs (Burke and Light, 1981). However, the superiority of recognition over recall is not in doubt. On the F-test the age deficit in recall is much larger than the age difference in recognition (Rabinowitz, 1984). A recognition deficit presumably means defective encoding whereas a recall deficit means defective retrieval. Since elderly people have problems of encoding, age differences in recognition tasks are to be expected.

A 'controlled-lag-recognition' task shows better scores for young adult subjects relative to elderly subjects. The subjects receive a long list of words, some of which are repeated at later points in the sequence and some are not. As each word is presented, subjects have to decide whether it is a repetition or a new word. The accuracy of performance in three groups, young, middle aged and old is respectively 93.9%, 80.8% and 76.4% (Rankin and Kausler, 1979). Elderly subjects are also impaired at retrieval of traces for prior conversation, in spite of the automaticity of incidental learning. The magnitude of age differences is higher for recall than for recognition. It has been suggested that a reduction in 'working memory' with age reduces the active search in the memory store and is thus responsible for this age-dependent memory problem (Kausler, 1985). Working memory is a cognitive structure with limited capacity that retains incoming information and maintains it like a scratch-pad memory for use in current processes. There is a good deal of evidence that it declines with age (e.g. Hasher and Zacks, 1979; Wright, 1981).

Multistore models and depth of processing theory

For many years, memory has been conceived as a set of different stores. According to the most common classification in frequent clinical use, storage is divided into short-term memory (STM) followed by long-term memory (LTM). STM has little capacity and the stored information is short-lived, but there is no effort in recall and the traces do not deteriorate so long as the materal is kept in mind by continuous use. On the other hand, LTM has an unmeasurable capacity and the information may be stored for a lifetime. However, recall is effortful and the recalled traces may be different from those encoded.

An elaboration of this dual-store model is the multistore-model. According to this, the first stage is a very-short-term- memory, the sensory buffer, followed by the primary memory (PM), memory for what is going on, secondary memory (SM), memory of unlimited capacity and duration, and finally tertiary memory (TM), memory for very old items. The age variations in this information-processing model are different: '(1) sensory memory, if not impaired, at least is not processed as efficiently in old age; (2) PM may hold up better, but (3) SM is clearly impaired; (4) TM may or may not hold up with age. (Botwinick, 1984.)

There is debate about the quality of episodic memory for events of long ago. It is worth considering the feeling of the Nobel prize winner Luigi Pirandello (1867–1936), who argues that we do not remember the past, although we believe we do:

"Is this the street? Is this the house? Is this the garden? Upon my visit after so many years to the small village where I was born and where I spent my infancy and my early adolescence, I realized that the place, albeit unchanged, was not the same one as was in me and my memories ... that life did not exist outside me. And now, facing the things — that are different because I was different — that life appeared unreal to me, like a dream."

In experimental research few papers deal with autobiographical research. A recent investigation does not consider that the accuracy of recall from the subject's past is really an issue, but the speed with which memories are reported and their distribution with age. Autobiographical memory has been studied in four groups, i.e. junior high, college, middle-aged and older adults. The main findings are the regularity and the stability in remembering patterns over the life span (Fitzgerald and Lawrence, 1984). The data are not at odds with laboratory research which mainly investigates episodic memory. Episodic memory requires effort, as in free or paired recall or in memory for prose and space. According to the difference between automatic and effortful functions (Hasher and Zacks, 1979), memory for daily events is more automatic. The stability of autobiographical events, albeit inaccurate, probably involves some 'semantic memory', i.e. memory for facts rather than for personal experience, which is thought to be age-independent.

An alternative view to the multistore model is the depth of processing model. For the purpose of perception and comprehension information is processed in two qualitatively different ways. One way is the 'shallow' level of analysis that processes sensory and physical patterns, the other way is the 'deep' level, which is involved in semantic, abstract and associative processes. Both mechanisms go on together, but primary memory is associated with more shallow processing and secondary memory with deeper processing. Elderly subjects fail to process deeply both at encoding and retrieval, but processing can be appropriately guided and practice reduces the effort (Craik and Simon, 1980). Shallow processing does not show age-difference under incidental conditions. Under intentional circumstances young subjects improve both shallow and deep processing, but elderly subjects show almost no improvement (Erber et al., 1980). The authors say that 'the old have more difficulty than the young in dealing with two instructional components simultaneously', an explanation compatible with the problem of attention tradeoff.

Metamemory

Metamemory is the knowledge of one's own memory ability ('how much can I learn, how much can I remember?'). There are some conflicting data on age-dependent changes in metamemory. It has recently been found that monitoring of the relative memorability of each of 60 word pairs shows no difference between elderly and young subjects, whereas from the total number of correct matches predicted, one can see that elderly subjects tend to overestimate their recall ability (Lovelace and Marsh, 1985), contrary to what might be expected.

Spatial abilities

There is a considerable amount of literature which indicates a decline in spatial abilities with age. For example, visualization, speed of closure and flexibility of closure (see Table 8.4 for explanation of terms) are affected, some of them showing an inverted V function over the life span (Horn and Cattell, 1967).

In the framework of effortful (age-sensitive) versus automatic (age-insensitive) processing, three brain functions are supposed to be carried out without any expenditure of effort, being 'genetically prepared', i.e. the frequency, time and

Table 8.4   Explanation of some psychological terms in this chapter

---

Backward masking = two tachistoscopically exposed stimuli are separated by a short time interval. Usually the first stimulus is a single letter (the target), whereas the second stimulus is a mask, which may disrupt the processing of the target stimulus.

Deep processing = the encoding of an item considers its meaning.

Episodic memory = the memory for personal experience.

Flexibility of closure = a primary mental ability (Horn, 1975), as measured in embedded figures (is a given geometrical figure embedded in a complex pattern?) and hidden pictures (find shapes and forms hidden in a drawing).

Frequency-of-occurrence = a subject is given a memory test, consisting for example of a lengthy series of words. At the end he will be asked about the frequency of certain words.

Incidental memory = a trace in memory without volitional effort (what did you eat last night?).

Lexical decision paradigm = the task is to decide whether a letter string is a word.

Orienting task = a mental activity to assure attention is directed at each list item (see deep and shallow processing).

Perceptual window = the elements which are seen at once when the subject stares at a display.

Priming = the processing of a given word is facilitated by a previous, semantically related word. An example of related, high dominance condition is the pair bird–robin, whereas the pair bird–duck is an example of related, low dominance condition.

Proactive inhibition = before learning, interference causes competition on recall.

Retroactive inhibition = after learning, interference causes competition on recall.

Shallow processing = non-semantic aspects are processed, such as the number of a given letter in a word or the search of a given initial.

Speed of closure = a primary mental ability (Horn, 1975), as measured in Gestalt completion (write the name of an object depicted only in part) and peripheral span (identify letters flashed in the periphery of the visual field).

Speed–accuracy tradeoff = the elderly are slower but more accurate.

Transfer = learning of a particular task is influenced by the previous learning of other tasks. It can be either positive or negative. The transfer can also be unspecific ('learning-to-learn' and 'warm-up'). In this case it is always positive.

Visualization = a primary mental ability (Horn, 1975), as measured in punched holes (how holes in folded paper would appear after paper is unfolded?) and clocks (how clock would look after having been rotated?).

---

place of occurrence. According to the Hasher–Zacks theory they should therefore not change with age. While frequency-of-occurrence and temporal information appear to be automatically processed in many experiments (see Botwinick, 1984), some data do not support the theory on the automatic processing of spatial information, since age-differences are found.

For example, psychometric test performance on memory for designs (Benton Revised Retention Test) declines with age, especially after age 70. But there is also the intriguing observation that this decline is not uniform, since in some elderly subjects it declines and in others it does not (Arenberg, 1978). In the same study, WAIS vocabulary performance shows small differences across the population, the older subjects slightly outscoring the young controls. This finding may indicate that spatial performance is not completely automatic, since a silent verbal reinforcement, such as geometrical tems, can occur. As a matter of fact, in a sequential mental rotation test where semi-abstract figures are rotated in two dimensions, older women improve their score through the use of meaningful labels. This finding indicates the usefulness of verbal strategy in spatial performance (Clarkson–Smith and Halpern, 1983).

Visual spatial learning is confirmed to be more sensitive to age than auditory verbal learning by other experiments on the spatial location of very familiar objects (Muramoto, 1984), although it can be argued that this task is not completely 'spatial' since verbal mediators, such as the objects' names, are certainly used by the subjects. Therefore, it is conceivable that what declines with age is the effective use of these mediators. In this case, the possibility of an automatic encoding of the true spatial component still exists.

In order to minimize the verbal component in a test of visual spatial memory, we studied the performance of two cohorts, with mean ages of 29 and 71, on the block tapping test (Fig. 8.5). The age-differences are very clear, although

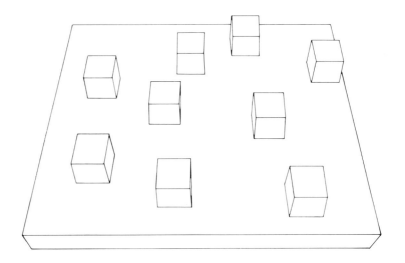

Fig. 8.5   Block tapping test. The white board is 25 × 20 cm. Each cube has a side of 2.5 cm

elderly subjects outscore deteriorated patients (Fig. 8.6). The mean scores are: controls 6.55 (s.d. 1.39), elderly 4.85 (s.d. 1.31), demented 1.13 (s.d 1.38). Although this test consists of nine identical white cubes and does not call for physical fitness and is free of cultural bias, silent verbal mediation cannot be completely ruled out, as for example 'up and down', 'left and right'. Other evidence for an age difference in processing of spatial information is provided by experiments on tactile learning (Moore et al., 1984). The data therefore weigh against the concept of automatic processing being independent of age. The automatic encoding of spatial locations is probably still an issue.

Mental rotation in tasks on matching rotated blocks shows not only age differences, but also sex differences at all ages, men being more accurate than women (Herman and Bruce, 1983). Other tests of spatial competence show a decline with age, for example visuospatial illusions, perspective-taking ability, spatial location and mental rotation (see Kirasic and Allen, 1985). Age differences in depicting and perceiving three-dimensionality have been seen (Plude

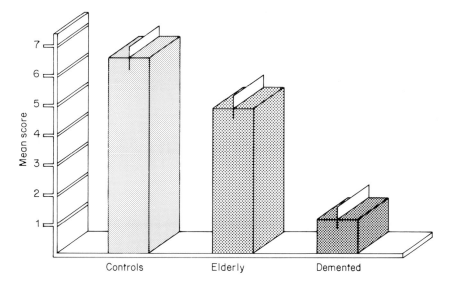

Fig. 8.6 Block tapping test. The three columns correspond to young controls (N = 100), normal elderly (N = 48) and demented subjects (N = 14)

et al., 1985). When elderly subjects draw solid cubes they are less accurate than young controls and are more prone to accept distorted cubes as accurate. Age-dependent changes are also seen, when mirror images in a task involving three-dimensional objects must be identified (Puglisi, 1985). This result confirms previous data on mental rotation with two-dimensional stimuli.

Again, laboratory tests have a number of limitations. These include cohort effects because young people are more used to driving and to be involved in sports like tennis or to the use of video games, which are high speed tests of spatial location. Effortful encoding can be shifted to automatic encoding by overlearning which therefore offsets the tradeoff in attention, when concomitant tasks place a high demand on mental abilities. Moreover, unfamiliar tasks can increase wariness in the elderly and a difficulty in understanding instructions can induce a conservative attitude to avoiding mistakes. Our experiments show that elderly subjects have no impairment in the recognition of clear and familiar patterns, but they are penalized on tasks in which the stimuli are ambiguous (Table 8.5). Elderly subjects show behavioural efficiency in a familiar and meaningful context, such as their grocery shopping, which is important in everyday life (Kirasic and

Allen, 1985). Conversely, the performance of young adults is not affected by the familiarity of the task setting. In another study no deficit is found for elderly relative to middle-aged subjects for intentional memory for the location of objects in a meaningful landscape; however, age deficits emerge when the location is in a random array (Waddell and Rogoff, 1981). Thus, no age variation is seen with a more ecological approach, that is to say, one which is closer to a real-life situation. This conclusion is also supported by studies of tasks involving locations either in a mock city or in locations within the subjects' home town. Age-

Table 8.5   Tachistoscopy for patterns (msec)

Group	Neat	Shading	Significance
Controls	18	28	
Elderly	18	639***	
Demented	2178***	5752***	***P < 0.001

	Accuracy		
Controls	100%	100%	
Elderly	100%	100%	
Demented	64%	64%	

dependent decline in performance only occurs in the former condition (Kirasic and Allen, 1985). However, where young people have a better elaborative strategy in recalling the urban environment (for example, description of buildings and spatial location), not only do elderly subjects have less knowledge of the urban landmarks, they are also less accurate in locating familiar buildings (Evans et al., 1984). Characteristics enhancing spatial information for elderly adults are displayed in Fig. 8.7.

Memory for movements shows changes similar to those found for other items, namely in capacity and efficiency. If 12 consecutive linear movements are encoded, young and old subjects have the same performance for immediate recall in the case of a small number of items, but age-dependent differences emerge when a higher requirement is called for by nine movements or more. In both groups, performance can be improved by organizational schemes imposed by the experimenter (Toole et al., 1984). As we shall see in Chapter 12, the tactual mode can be helpful for the assimilation of motor patterns, although tactual stimuli have been reported to be remembered less well by elderly subjects (Riege and Inman, 1981).

Work activity is certainly an important factor in favouring automatic encoding of spatial location. Thus a taxi driver will be more highly trained than a diplomat in spatial skills. Matching subjects on the basis of age and years of education in psychometric research may not rule out a bias in composition of the groups.

A greater decline of spatial abilities compared to verbal ones might lead to the conclusion of a selective aging process affecting the right hemisphere. This conclusion is ruled out by neuropsychological observations (Caltagirone and Benedetti, 1983; Nebes et al., 1983; Byrd and Moscovitch, 1984; Obler et al.,

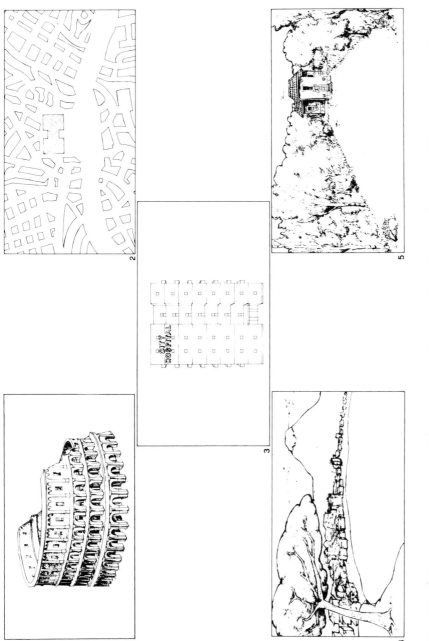

Fig. 8.7 Building characteristics which enhance spatial orientation. Historical landmarks (1), direct access (2), 'use intensity' (3), natural landscaping (4) and siting characteristics (5) provide elderly people with cues for spatial orientation. Evans et al., 1984, freely interpreted

1984). Moreover, as we saw in the previous chapter, many electrophysiological data do not support the view of programmed asymmetrical aging.

LANGUAGE

There is a good deal of evidence that verbal abilities are stable over the life span. Verbal functioning should not be thought of as restricted to the left hemisphere only, because visual imagery and functions involving the right hemisphere are certainly brought into play when a person is involved in the use of language. Overlearning, familiar context and professional experience are certainly contributory factors to the stability of language over the years.

The pioneering studies on cognitive aging recognized that verbal abilities tend to decline very little, or not at all, with age. In this respect language differs from perceptual-integrative skills particularly when speed of response is required. Primary mental abilities in the framework of so-called crystallized intelligence even display an increase during the period that 'fluid intelligence' decreases (Horn, 1975). The types of performance which survive best involve verbal comprehension, general information, associative fluency and ideational fluency, that is to say unpaced tasks.

In tasks of lexical decision, semantic priming (Table 8.4) is preserved in late life, regardless of whether the words are category-member (e.g. rain–snow) or descriptive-property associates (e.g. rain–wet). Probably a spread of automatic age-independent semantic activation is involved. In the word–nonword condition (e.g. dollar–quibe) the young subjects may have a worse performance, because they may take a decision too fast on the basis of the first word (Howard et al., 1981). While the encoding of random letters slows down by 20 or 30% with age, the time required to recover a meaningful word, and semantic associations between words, is considered to be unaffected by age (Cerella and Fozard, 1984). However, Madden (1985) found a slight age effect on semantic retrieval time, which is 259 msec for the young adults and 352 msec for the elderly subjects. Free recall of words in the Auditory Verbal Learning Test is similar in two cohorts with median ages of 40 and 60 (Bleecker et al., 1985). Similar learning curves, but different intercepts have been found by us in two groups, with mean ages of 29 and 40; demented patients have quite a diffferent pattern (Fig. 8.8). The sparing of linguistic function with age is an important argument against the interpretation of dementia as exaggerated aging (Gainotti et al., 1980; Goldstein, 1980; Emery, 1985).

The first longitudinal study, the Iowa State Study, has indicated stability or even improvement in vocabulary (Fig. 8.9) and recent studies support the hypothesis of age stability in vocabulary test performance (O'Dowd, 1983). Elderly subjects give more synonyms and can compensate for a 'warm up' bias by their better knowledge of difficult items at the end of the WAIS vocabulary subtest. Stability has also been seen in a longitudinal study using a different vocabulary test, where 50 male subjects ranging from 60 to 79 years of age were examined three times (Poitrenaud et al., 1983). In this study, contrary to other tests exploring 'fluid intelligence', performance on the vocabulary test was stable until at least age 75–80 (see also Fig. 8.10).

Elderly subjects show as much semantic priming as young adults and a similar number of errors (without a speed–accuracy tradeoff), but are impaired on recall and recognition of the words (Howard, 1983). The prime effect is the response time on unrelated word pairs minus response time on related trials; for both groups of subjects the lowest time is scored with related, high dominance items (Table 8.4).

No difference is seen between young and elderly subjects in the accuracy of

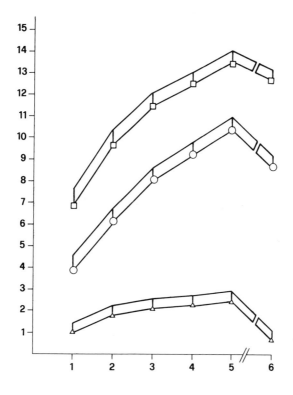

REY VERBAL TEST

Fig. 8.8 Free recall and delayed recall from a list of 15 familiar words in three groups, young (□, N = 100), older adults (○, N = 48) and demented subjects (△, N = 14). The elderly and the control subjects have the same slope and a different intercept. Y-axis: recalled words. X-axis: trials. For each trial $p < 0.01$. The demented group differ both in intercept and in slope

lexical decision, although the elderly respond more slowly; the longer latency is dependent on a retrieval deficit in semantic memory processing (Bowles and Poon, 1985). This stability in semantic priming occurs both under automatic and controlled (effortful) information processing (Chiarello et al., 1985).

The semantic processing of sentences and the access to implied information do not change with age, although elderly subjects are less able to recognize details of the sentence. Age-deficits in comprehension may be spurious, since the techniques used evaluate what the elderly person remembers rather than what he has understood (Burke and Yee, 1984). In the elderly the conceptual trend is to go from abstract to concrete dimensions of categorization, while the opposite is true in children (Howard, 1983). Sensitivity to the relative importance of information is stable with age in spite of decreased recall (Surber et al., 1984). Semantic

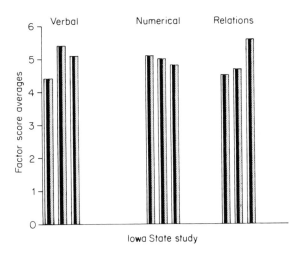

Fig. 8.9 Iowa Longitudinal Study. The estimated factor scores were averaged over 96 subjects across three occasions of measurements: 1919, 1950, 1961. The verbal factor score has a significant increment from the first to the second occasion of measurement. The numerical factor shows a significant decrement from the second to the third occasion. Adapted from Cunningham and Owens, 1983, with permission

information processing seems therefore to be qualitatively stable over the life span, but the speed of semantic judgement is lower in the elderly (Raskind et al., 1985). When a story has to be remembered, elderly people recall the gist like the young, but they are less able to recall details and to comprehend stories which were rearranged and so are no longer well ordered (Mandel, 1985). It is not clear yet whether the older subjects do not remember discourse as well as young adults on account of age differences in the storage and manipulation of information by working memory (Light and Anderson, 1985). An alternative explanation is the difficulty in sustained attention as indicated by experiments on the CNV (see the previous chapter).

Cued recall shows no age differences when the cuing is controlled to ensure that all subjects use the same type of processing, i.e. when the word list is composed of 'instances of common conceptual categories and the search criterion is based on category membership. That is, the subject would have to search for a tool in the list (e.g., hammer), then an animal (e.g., elephant) and so on'. Under these conditions the category labels are used as cues for recall (Macht and Buschke, 1984).

When we move to the higher stages of the comprehension process, such as the integration of sentences into discourse and the generation of inferences, we are faced with ambiguous evidence, which is probably of little general validity. Thinking is not a unitary function. Not only is it certainly affected by age but also by ethnic and historic factors. For example, the prose, poetry and articles in newspapers of the last century are certainly very different from what is written today. Construction of African languages is certainly different from English, and Latin syntax differs from that of Sanskrit. Since discourse processors are still largely undefined, there is a lack of theory on complex linguistic behaviour. According to a recent review, 'we have not arrived yet at schedules and plans; the effortful encoding of a list of names is a typical laboratory task, that differs from most of those in everyday life and normal conversation' (Kausler, 1982).

The quality of encoding is also affected by a variety of other factors. Since the cognitive effort required for rehearsal processes is considered to be the source of age deficits in the encoding of information (Kausler, 1985), picture recognition improves in tasks which allow interim rehearsal (Harker and Riege, 1985). Older adults also improve their memory performance if they are allowed to participate in the initial determination of what is to be remembered, where they elaborate encoding through self-generation of rhymes and synonyms of stimulus words (McFarland et al., 1985). Time constraints are known to affect encoding. While the comprehension of a meaningful discourse and the ability to make logical inferences from it are not lost with age, an impairment is seen at high speeds of presentation (Stine et al., 1985). The limitation here is probably accounted for by the stimulus–persistence hypothesis, since the speech sounds must be 'cleared through the nervous system'. A high stimulus presentation rate therefore impairs encoding in the elderly, which in turn worsens any pre-existing difficulty in organization of the items to be remembered (e.g. Sanders et al., 1980). However, if orienting tasks are added to constrain encoding to relevant stimuli, the age difference is reduced (Craik and Rabinowitz, 1985). On the other hand the authors find that a slower presentation rate helps young subjects to carry out more processing operations and therefore increases the age difference. In a memory task elderly subjects recalled fewer words than younger controls and their recall was less affected by orienting task instructions, such as phonological or semantic (Rankin and Hyland, 1983). Young subjects greatly improve their free recall performance if they receive congruent orienting, unlike elderly subjects. Cued recall under these conditions improves performance in both groups (Erber, 1984).

Anxiety interferes with performance in a face–name test among elderly subjects. Training which improves relaxation improves recall because it favours a better attention (Yesavage and Jacob, 1984). Supporting and encouraging contexts (i.e., 'Please, help me') are more helpful than challenging ones (i.e. 'Show me your ability') and self-generated verbal or image mediators also seem to facilitate encoding in the elderly (see Botwinick, 1984), although to a lesser extent than in young controls. The use of imagery aims to relate items, such as those of a paired associated learning. These subjects are better able to develop mnemonic solutions to the problems which beset them. 'Life span changes in discourse operations are like a tantalus; the behaviour is observable but the key to understanding this change is still as elusive as ever' (Spilich, 1985).

The comprehension of sentences can be normal and yet memory for inferred information is reduced among elderly subjects, which appears to indicate that the deficit is in retrieval. Young, but not elderly adults can take advantage of their own associative reponses provided as cues (Perlmutter, 1979). An encoding task where elderly subjects have to decide about pleasantness of a sentence is performed less efficiently than a comprehension task, in contrast to young subjects, because the former are less likely to integrate the meaning of each sentence. Thus, a deficit in encoding is also suggested for age differences in inferential memory (Till, 1985).

PROBLEM SOLVING

Problem solving is a daily mental activity in both unfamiliar and familiar domains. Cashing a cheque at a bank or setting a meal are familiar activities for the elderly, whereas mastering new logical problems might be unfamiliar. In either case, a strategy must be searched for reaching the goal, starting from known data. Elderly people might be expected to have more difficulties with these strategies, which call for high memory load and speed of processing. Working memory has a low capacity and is not so keen in old age as in youth (e.g., Hasher and Zacks, 1979; Wright, 1981; Welford, 1985) with the result that problems arise in storage and processing. On the other hand, performance in virtually all forms of employment and professional activity shows no decline with age, and is even supposed to improve in certain cases. The middle aged perform better than the young in practical problem solving tasks that call for experience. However, in spite of attempts to bias problems in favour of elderly subjects, they do not outperform younger adults. Aging effects are therefore not offset by increased experience (Denney and Pearce, 1985).

Chess and bridge provide unusual opportunities to investigate problem solving in the elderly in an ecologically valid context. Since these games are played today with the same rules as 100 years ago, they do not encounter significant cohort effects. Although aging affects performance in the two games in somewhat different ways, the general conclusions are that: (1) there is no decline with age; and (2) previous experience is much more important than age (Charness, 1985). This author states that 'as bridge players and chess players age, they may become slower at encoding information about the problem, but once the problem space has been represented, they search it as effectively as their level of acquired skill permits'. Such findings should not be taken to mean that the psychometric evidence for memory loss is artifactual; it is, however, situation-specific. Although recall is known to worsen with age, older players recall more cards with a one second exposure than do unskilled young subjects with a longer exposure. An important conclusion is drawn once more from these studies: variance among elderly people is high, especially when education plays a role in performance. When subjects are equated for educational levels or when a familiar setting is used, age differences are reduced or vanish.

PERSONALITY

Young people quickly react to sudden external changes, while the elderly are apt to respond with more cautious behaviour. The conservative attitude as a source of bias has been widely reported in neuropsychology. The young act as innovators, the aged as a 'cultural anchor' (Mergler and Goldstein, quoted by Spilich, 1985). A saying has it that 'we are born as fire-raisers and die as fire-men'.

However, longitudinal studies (LS), like the Bonn LS, do not confirm the existence of such stereotypes in old age. A high variability in personality patterns does not permit any general theory. This study reports different kinds of self-perception: one group, for example, does not complain of changes in health, occupation, mental abilities and social life, whereas another reports an above-average list of complaints (Schmitz-Scherzer and Thomae, 1983). However, over the whole period of study, the highest score for reported stress and reactions to stress involves health problems. Problems concerning vision, hearing and mobility are more frequent in the older subjects.

The same conclusions are drawn by the Baltimore LS (Costa et al., 1983). Consistency over time of individual differences and mean levels of disposition indicate that variations in personality are age independent. The stability of personality gives a contribution to the coherence and continuity in the individual's life because stability in personality and self, coupled with maintenance of roles and relationships with the environment, constitutes a defensive mechanism against negative inputs to the self-image (Atchley, 1982).

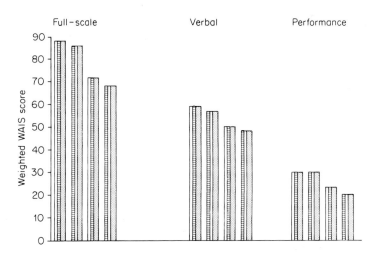

Fig. 8.10   Duke Longitudinal Study. WAIS performance as a function of distance from death. For each group of tests (full-scale, verbal and performance) the distance is grouped in four bands (from left to right): 15–19, 10–14, 5–9 and 0–4 years. The change in full-scale scores as a function of distance from death is statistically significant. 76% of the sample decline before death. Adapted from Siegler, 1983, with permission

The Duke LS also shows remarkable stability of personality patterns and some data indicate that 76% of the sample has a terminal cognitive decline (Siegler, 1983). Fig. 8.10 displays WAIS performance as a function of distance from death.

Recent research on a Swedish sample (Nilsson and Persson, 1983) confirms that personality dimensions change little from age 70 to age 79. In men a slight decrease of emotional involvement is observed, and in women, more cautious behaviour in avoiding new and difficult tasks. Between 75 and 79 it is reported that there is an increase in changeability, impulsiveness and suggestibility, which are not attributed by the authors to any organic syndrome like the so-called 'preterminal drop'. The magnitude of individual variability and sex differences do not change.

A different kind of longitudinal study stems from observations at Bell System, the large American company. The group covered by this project, called the Management Process Study, is not representative of the general population since the study was aimed at the identification of factors determining the qualities of good managers, such as age, personal history and experience, and their changes with age (Bray and Howard, 1983). It is reported that corporation, i.e. belonging to a large industrial company, does not produce clones and overwhelm personality. On the contrary, it enhances the differences in personality. Moreover age changes in managerial ability are related to success on the job. Decline with age is very clear among those who had low managerial ability, low motivation and poor advancement.

TESTING THE ELDERLY

There is a tendency for the various laboratories to use their own methodologies. A pertinent review of this problem is introduced by a witty remark reminding the reader of the tower of Bable (Israel et al., 1984). In this work one-, two- and three-dimensional measurements are collected, i.e. those which measure mental, mental + physical, mental + physical + social variables.

Of the 84 one-dimensional measurements alone, 19 deal with emotions and affective behaviour, 47 deal with cognitive functions and 18 concern measurements of general behaviour. Which is to be used?

Amid so much diversity, the need for precise methodology is clear. No definite conclusions can be reached without agreement on research protocols. These must allow the quantification of cognitive loss and provide an indication of the probability of dementia in each case. Many of the batteries are too global, often based on interview or open-ended questions. Self-rating errs on the side of excess (Raskin, 1979). In the field of intelligence Wechsler himself pointed out that his test was not applicable to the elderly. The first question we have to ask ourselves is 'to whom' does a test apply? (Plutchik, 1979). The elderly need batteries that are relevant to them, which interest them, and which are not too tedious but call for quick responses reflecting the demands of modern life in the urban environment (Crook, 1979).

It is important to select subjects for research projects with care. Some studies include subjects in their 50s among the elderly. Medication is seldom reported in neuropsychological articles, although the extensive use of tranquillizers among the elderly is well known. These drugs affect mental operations, especially paced ones and so they may interfere with the results. Electrophysiological research is more reliable in this respect, because such drugs certainly affect the EEG and so reveal the presence of inhomogeneity in the group.

We feel that since the operations of the neuronal network are timed in milliseconds, we need tests which explore the processing of simple tasks with the smallest number of variables and which express the result as an objective physiological measure and not in some arbitrary form like a rating scale. For this reason we are in favour of a cognitive microanalysis (Eisdorfer and Cohen, 1982) with laboratory tests specifically designed for the study of one or more functions in order to test particular information processing operations and specialized cerebral structures. A recent conference on Alzheimer's disease concluded that: 'illiterate subjects, or persons from different cultures might perform poorly on a cognitive test, not because of illness and disability but because of the difficulty and inappropriateness of the test procedures. Tests of first-order capabilities such as visual perception, reaction time, or motor ability might be closer to measuring substrate levels of (CNS) integrity and disability without the complication of trying to measure abstract–conceptual–cognitive behaviour' (Khachaturian, 1985).

Testing the elderly subject is important not just for research but for routine clinical diagnosis of Alzheimer's disease, in order to obtain normative data. In the previous chapter several electrophysiological measures were shown to be useful in differentiating aging from dementia. Neurophysiological batteries are also valuable for this purpose. For example, cluster analysis on tests of first order capabilities, such as those just indicated, differentiates three groups, respectively young controls, old normal adults and demented patients with 86% accuracy (Giaquinto et al., 1985). Another battery including verbal tasks (token test, verbal fluency, memory for prose) and non-verbal tasks (finger agnosia, constructional apraxia, sorting test) misclassifies 20% of demented patients and 10% of normal subjects (Bandera et al., 1985).

As we shall see in Chapter 12, rigorous methods of testing are also needed to evaluate and improve neuropsychological training techniques for the maintenance and rehabilitation of elderly subjects.

REFERENCES

Amberson, J. I., Atkenson, B. M., Pollack, R. H., and Malatesta, V. J. (1979). Age differences in dark-interval threshold across the life-span. *Exp. Aging Res.*, 5, 423–433.

Arenberg, D. (1978). Differences and changes with age in the Benton visual retention test. *J. Gerontol.*, 33, 534–540.

Atchley, R. C. (1982). The aging self. *Psychotherapy*, 19, 388–396.

Bandera, R., Capitani, E., Della Sala, S., and Spinnler, H. (1985). Discrimination between senile dementia Alzheimer type patients and education matched normal controls by means of a 6-test set. *Ital. J. Neurol. Sci.*, 6, 339–344.

Barrett, T. R., and Wright, M. (1981). Age-related facilitation in recall following semantic processing. *J. Gerontol.*, 2., 194–199.

Birren, J. (1974). Psychophysiology and speed of response. *Amer. Psychol.*, 29, 808–815.
Birren, J. E., Cunningham, W. R., and Yamamoto, K. (1983). Psychology of adult development and aging. *Ann. Rev. Psychol.*, 34, 543–575.
Bleecker, M. L., Bolla-Wilson, K., and Heller, J. R. (1985). The effect of aging on learning curves. *Ann N.Y. Acad. Sci.*, 444, 499–501.
Botwinick, J. (1978). *Aging and Behaviour* (2nd Ed.). New York: Springer.
Botwinick, J. (1984). *Aging and Behaviour.* New York: Springer Publ. Co.
Bowles, N. L., and Poon, L. W. (1985). Aging and retrieval of words in semantic memory. *J. Gerontol.*, 40, 71–77.
Bray, D. W., and Howard, A. (1983). The AT&T longitudinal studies of managers. In K. W. Schaie (Ed.), *Longitudinal Studies of Adult Psychological Development.* New York: The Guildford Press, pp. 266–312.
Burke, D. M., and Light, L. L. (1981). Memory and aging: the role of retrieval processes. *Psychol. Bull.*, 90, 513–546.
Burke, D. M., and Yee, P. L. (1984). Semantic priming during sentence processing by young and older adults. *Dev. Psychol.*, 20, 903–910.
Byrd, M., and Moscovitch, M. (1984). Lateralization of peripherally and centrally masked words in young and elderly people. *J. Gerontol.*, 39, 699–703.
Caltagirone, C., and Benedetti, N. (1983). L'invecchiamento produce un decremento asimmetrico delle prestazioni intellettive mediate dai due emisferi cerebrali? *Arch. Psicol. Neurol. Psichiatr.*, 44, 336–348.
Cavanaugh, J. C. (1983). Comprehension and retention of television programs by 20- and 60-year olds. *J. Gerontol.*, 38, 190–196.
Cerella, J. (1985). Age-related decline in extrafoveal letter perception. *J. Gerontol.*, 40, 727–736.
Cerella, J., and Fozard, J. L. (1984). Lexical access and age. *Dev. Psychol.*, 20, 235–243.
Cerella, J., Poon, L. W., and Fozard, J. L. (1982). Age and iconic read-out. *J. Gerontol.*, 37, 197–202.
Cerella, J., Poon, L. W., and Williams, D. M. (1980). Age and the complexity hypothesis. In L. W. Poon (Ed.), *Aging in the 1980's: Psychological Issues.* Washington, D.C.: American Psychological Association, pp. 332–340.
Charness, N. (1985). Aging and problem solving performance. In N. Charness (Ed.), *Aging and Human Performance.* New York: John Wiley & Sons, pp. 225–259.
Chiarello, C., Church, K. L., and Hoyer, W. J. (1985). Automatic and controlled semantic priming: accuracy, response bias, and aging. *J. Gerontol.*, 40, 593–600.
Clarkson-Smith, L., and Halpern, D. F. (1983). Can age-related deficits in spatial memory be attenuated through the use of verbal coding? *Exp. Aging Res.*, 9, 179–184.
Cohen, G., and Faulkner, D. (1983). Word recognition: age differences in contextual facilitation effects. *Brit. J. Psychol.*, 74, 239–251.
Costa, Jr., P. T., McCrae, R. R., and Arenberg, D. (1983). Recent longitudinal research on personality and aging. In K. W. Schaie (Ed.), *Longitudinal Studies of Adult Psychological Development.* New York: The Guildford Press, pp. 222–265.
Craik, F. I. M., and Rabinowitz, J. C. (1985). The effects of presentation rate and encoding task on age-related memory deficits. *J. Gerontol.*, 40, 309–315.
Craik, F. I. M., and Simon, E. (1980). Age differences in memory: the role of attention and depth of processing. In L. W. Poon, J. L. Fozard, L. S. Cermak, D. Arenberg and L. W. Thompson (Eds), *New Direction in Memory and Aging.* Hillsdale N.J.: Erlbaum, pp. 95–112.
Crook, T. H. (1979). Psychometric assessment in the elderly. In A. Raskin and L. F. Jarvik (Eds), *Psychiatric Symptoms and Cognitive Loss in the Elderly.* New York: John Wiley & Sons, 207–220.
Cunningham, W. R. (1980) Speed, age and qualitative differences in cognitive functioning. In L. W. Poon (Ed.), *Aging in the 1980's: Psychological Issues.* Washington DC: American Psychological Association, pp. 327–331.

Cunningham, W. R., and Owens Jr., W. A. (1983). The Iowa State Study of the adult development of intellectual abilities. In K. W. Schaie (Ed.), *Longitudinal Studies of Adult Psychological Development*. New York: The Guildford Press, pp. 20–39.

Denney, N. W., and Pearce, K. A. (1985). Practical problem solving in elderly adults. *Gerontologist*, 25, 166.

Eisdorfer, C., and Cohen, D. (1982). The assessment of organic impairment in the aged. In E. I. Burdock, A. Sudilovski and S. Gershon (Eds), *The Behaviour of Psychiatric Patients*. New York: Dekker, pp. 329–351.

Emery, O. B. (1985). Language and aging. *Exp. Aging Res.*, 11, 3–60.

Erber, J., Herman, T. G., and Botwinick, J. (1980). Age differences in memory as a function of depth of processing. *Exp. Aging. Res.*, 6, 341–348.

Erber, J. T. (1984). Age differences in the effect of encoding congruence on incidental free and cued recall. *Exp. Aging Res.*, 10, 221–224.

Evans, G. W., Brennan, P. L., Skorpanich, M. A., and Held, D. (1984). Cognitive mapping and elderly adults: verbal and location memory for urban landmarks. *J. Gerontol.*, 39, 452–457.

Falk, J. L., and Kline, D. W. (1978). Stimulus persistence in CFF: overarousal or underactivation? *Exp. Aging Res.*, 4, 109–123.

Farkas, M. S., and Hoyer, W. J. (1980). Processing consequences of perceptual grouping in selective attention. *J. Gerontol.*, 35, 207–216.

Ferris, S. H., Crook, T., Clark, E., McCarthy, M., and Rae, D. (1980). Facial recognition memory deficits in normal aging and senile dementia. *J. Gerontol.*, 35, 707–714.

Fitzgerald, J. M., and Lawrence, R. (1984). Autobiographical memory across the life-span. *J. Gerontol.*, 39, 692–698.

Gainotti, G., Caltagirone, C., Masullo, G., and Miceli, G. (1980). Patterns of neuropsychological impairment in various diagnostic groups of dementia. In L. Amaducci, A. N. Davison and P. Antuono (Eds), *Aging*, vol. 13. New York: Raven Press, pp. 245–250.

Giaquinto, S., Nolfe, G., and Calvani, M. (1985). Cluster analysis of cognitive performance in elderly and demented subjects. *Ital. J. Neurol. Sci.*, 6, 157–165.

Gilmore, J. C., Tobias, T. R., and Royer, F. L. (1985). Aging and similarity grouping in visual search. *J. Gerontol.*, 40, 586–592.

Goldstein, G. (1980). Psychopathological dysfunction in the elderly: discussion. In J. O. Cole and J. E. Barrett (Eds), *Psychopathology in the Aged*. New York: Raven Press, pp. 137–144.

Gottsdanker, R. (1982). Age and simple reaction time. *J. Gerontol.*, 37, 342–348.

Gottsdanker, R. (1984). Effort of preparation and age. *Percept. Motor Skill*, 59, 527–538.

Hanley-Dunn, P., and McIntosh, J. L. (1984). Meaningfulness and recall of names by young and old adults. *J. Gerontol.*, 39, 583–585.

Harker, J. O., and Riege, W. H. (1985). Aging and delay effects on recognition of words and designs. *J. Gerontol.*, 40, 601–604.

Hasher, L., and Zacks, R. T. (1979). Automatic and effortful processes in memory. *J. Exp. Psychol.: General*, 108, 356–388.

Herman, J. F., and Bruce, P. R. (1983). Adults' mental rotation of spatial information: effects of age, sex and cerebral laterality. *Exp. Aging Res.*, 9, 83–85.

Hess, T. M. (1985). Effects of semantically related and unrelated contexts on recognition memory of different-aged adults. *J. Gerontol.*, 39, 444–451.

Hines, T. (1979). Information feedback, reaction time and error rates in young and old subjects. *Exp. Aging Res.*, 5, 207–215.

Horn, J. L. (1975). Psychometric studies of aging and intelligence. In S. Gershon, and A. Raskin (Eds), *Aging*, vol. 2. New York: Raven Press, pp. 19–43.

Horn, J. L., and Cattell, R. B. (1967). Age differences in fluid and crystallized intelligence. *Acta Psychol.*, 26, 107–129.

Howard, D. A., McAndrews, M. P., and Lasaga, M. I. (1981). Semantic priming of lexical decisions in young and old adults. *J. Gerontol.*, 36, 707–714.

Howard, D. V. (1983). The effects of aging and degree of association on the semantic priming of lexical decision. *Exp. Aging Res.*, 9, 145–151.

Israel, L., Kozarevic, D., and Sartorius, N. (1984). *Evaluations en Gérontologie*. Basel: Karger.

Kausler, D. H. (1982). *Experimental Psychology and Human Aging*. New York: John Wiley & Sons.

Kausler, D. H. (1985). Episodic memory: memorizing performance. In N. Charness (Ed.), *Aging and Human Performance*. New York: John Wiley & Sons, pp. 101–141.

Khachaturian, Z. S. (1985). Diagnosis of Alzheimer's disease. *Arch. Neurol.*, 42, 1097–1105.

Kirasic, K. C., and Allen, G. L. (1985). Aging, spatial performance and spatial competence. In N. Charness (Ed.), *Aging and Human Performance*. New York: John Wiley & Sons, pp. 191–223.

Kline, D. W. (1984). Processing sense information. In J. Botwinick (Ed.), *Aging and Behavior*. New York: Springer Publ. Co., pp. 207–228.

Kline, D. W., and Orme-Rogers, C. (1978). Examination of stimulus persistence as the basis for superior visual identification performance among older adults. *J. Gerontol.*, 33, 76–81.

Light, L. L., and Anderson, P. A. (1985). Working-memory capacity, age, and memory for discourse. *J. Gerontol.*, 40, 737–747.

Lovelace, E. A., and Marsh, G. R. (1985). Prediction and evaluation of memory performance by young and old adults. *J. Gerontol.*, 40, 192–197.

Macht, M. L., and Buschke, H. (1984). Speed of recall in aging. *J. Gerontol.*, 39, 439–443.

Madden, D. J. (1984). Data-driven and memory driven selective attention in visual search. *J. Gerontol.*, 39, 72–78.

Madden, D. J. (1985). Age-related slowing in the retrieval of information from long-term memory. *J. Gerontol.*, 40, 208–210.

Madden, D. J., and Nebes, R. D. (1980). Aging and the development of automaticity in visual search. *Dev. Psychol.*, 16, 377–384.

Mandel, R. G. (1985). Effects of age, story organization and number of presentation on recall of complex stories. *Gerontologist*, 25, 145.

Margolis, R. B., and Scialfa, C. T. (1984). Age differences in Wechsler memory scale performance. *J. Clin. Psychol.*, 40, 1442–1449.

McCormack, P. D. (1984). Aging and recognition memory: methodological and interpretative problems. *Exp. Aging Res.*, 10, 215–219.

McFarland jr, C. E., Warren, L. R., and Crockard, J. (1985). Memory of self-generated stimuli in young and old adults. *J. Gerontol.*, 40, 205–207.

Moore, T. E., Richards, B. and Hood, J. (1984). Aging and the coding of spatial information. *J. Gerontol.*, 39, 210–212.

Muramoto, O. (1984). Selective reminding in normal and demented aged people: auditory verbal versus visual spatial task. *Cortex*, 20, 461–478.

Nebes, R. D. (1978). Vocal versus manual response as a determinant of age difference in simple reaction time. *J. Gerontol.*, 33, 884–889.

Nebes, R. D., Madden, D. J., and Berg, W. D. (1983). The effect of age on hemispheric asymmetry in visual and auditory identification. *Exp. Aging Res.*, 9, 87–91.

Nilsson, L. V., and Pearson, G. (1983). Personality changes in the aged. *Acta Psychiatr. scand.*, 68, 414–418.

Nissen, M. J., and Corkin, S. (1985). Effectiveness of attentional cueing in older and younger adults. *J. Gerontol.*, 40, 185–191.

O'Dowd, S. C. (1983). Vocabulary test performance of old and young adults: another look at quality scoring. *J. Gen. Psychol.*, 109, 167–180.

Obler, L. K., Woodward, S., and Albert, M. L. (1984). Changes in cerebral lateralization in aging? *Neuropsychologia*, 22, 235–240.

Park, D. C., and Puglisi, J. T. (1985). Older adults' memory for the color of pictures and words. *J. Gerontol.*, 40, 198–204.

Perlmutter, M. (1979). Age differences in adults' free recall, cued recall, and recognition. *J. Gerontol.*, 34, 533–539.

Plude, D. J., and Hoyer, W. J. (1985). Attention and performance: identifying and localizing age deficits. In N. Charness (Ed.), *Aging and Human Performance*. New York: John Wiley & Sons, pp. 47–99.

Plude, D. J., Millberg, W. P., and Cerella, J. (1985). Age differences in depicting and perceiving tridimensionality. *Gerontologist*, 25, 201.

Plutchik, R. (1979). Conceptual and practical issues in the assessment of the elderly. In A. Raskin and L. F. Jarvik (Eds), *Psychiatric Symptoms and Cognitive Loss in the Elderly*. New York: John Wiley & Sons, pp. 19–38.

Poitrenaud, J., Barrère, H., Darcet, P., and Driss, F. (1983). Le viellissement des fonctions cognitives. *Presse Mèd.*, 48, 3119–3123.

Puglisi, J. T. (1985). Age related slowing in mental rotation of three-dimensional objects. *Gerontologist*, 25, 201.

Rabbitt, P. M. A. (1977). Changes in problem solving ability in old age. In J. E. Birren and K. W. Schaie (Eds), *Handbook of the Psychology of Aging*. New York: Van Nostrand Reinhold, pp. 606–625.

Rabinowitz, J. C. (1984). Aging and recognition failure. *J. Gerontol.*, 39, 65–71.

Rankin, J. L., and Collins, M. (1985). Adult age differences in memory elaboration. *J. Gerontol.*, 40, 451–458.

Rankin, J. L., and Hyland, T. P. (1983). The effects of orienting tasks on adult age differences in recall and recognition. *Exp. Aging Res.*, 9, 159–164.

Rankin, J. L., and Kausler, D. H. (1979). Adult age differences in false recognitions. *J. Gerontol.*, 34, 58–65.

Raskin, A. (1979). Signs and symptoms of psychotherapy in the elderly. In A. Raskin and L. F. Jarvik (Eds), *Psychiatric Symptoms and Cognitive Loss in the Elderly*. New York: John Wiley & Sons, pp. 3–18.

Raskind, C. L., Cannon, C. J., and Hertzog, C. (1985). Age-related slowing in the speed of semantic information processing. *Gerontologist*, 25, 204–205.

Riege, W. H., and Inman, V. (1981). Age differences in non-verbal memory tasks. *J. Gerontol.*, 36, 51–58.

Rissenberg, M. (1985). Identification of incomplete picture: the effects of normal aging and senile dementia of the Alzheimer's type. *Gerontologist*, 25, 74.

Salthouse, T. (1985). *A theory of Cognitive Aging*. Amsterdam: North-Holland.

Salthouse, T. A., and Lichty, W. (1985). Tests of the neural noise hypothesis of age-related cognitive change. *J. Gerontol.*, 40, 443–450.

Salthouse, T. A., and Somberg, B. L. (1982a). Isolating the age deficit in speeded performance. *J. Gerontol.*, 37, 59–63.

Salthouse, T. A., and Somberg, B. L. (1982b). Time-accuracy relationship in young and old adults. *J. Gerontol.*, 37, 349–353.

Sanders, R. E., Murphy, R. D., Schmitt, F. A., and Walsh, K. K. (1980). Age differences in free recall rehearsal strategies. *J. Gerontol.*, 35, 550–558.

Schmitt, F. O., Dev, P., and Smith, B. H. (1976). Electrotonic processing of information by brain cells. *Science*, 193, 114–120.

Schmitz–Scherzer, R., and Thomae, H. (1983). Constancy and change of behavior in old age: findings from the Bonn Longitudinal Study on aging. In K. W. Schaie (Ed.), *Longitudinal Studies of Adult Psychological Development*. New York: The Guildford Press, pp. 191–221.

Siegler, I. C. (1983). Psychological aspects of the Duke Longitudinal Studies. In K. W. Schaie (Ed.), *Longitudinal Studies of Adult Psychological Development*. New York: The Guildford Press, pp. 137–190.

Simon, J. R., and Pouraghabagher, A. R. (1978). The effect of aging on the stages of processing in a choice reaction time task. *J. Gerontol.*, 33, 553–561.

Smith, A. D. (1980). Age differences in encoding, storage, and retrieval. In L. W. Poon, J. L. Fozard, L. S. Cermak, D. Arenberg and L. W. Thompson (Eds), *New Directions in Memory and Aging*. Hillsdale: Lawrence Erlbaum Ass., pp. 23–46.

Smith, G. A., and Brewer, N. (1985). Age and individual differences in correct and error reaction times. *Brit. J. Psychiat.*, 76, 199–203.

Smith, M. C., Greeley, H., Roberts-DeRoo T., and Reeves, A. G. (1985). Central reaction time in normal aging. *Ann. Neurol.*, 18, 145–146.

Spilich, G. J. (1985). Discourse comprehension across the span of life. In N. Charness (Ed.), *Aging and Human Performance*. New York: John Wiley & Sons, pp. 143–190.

Stine, E. L., Wingfield, A., and Poon, L. W. (1985). Speech comprehension among elderly adults of average and above-average verbal ability. *Gerontologist*, 25, 144.

Surber, J. R., Kowalski, A. H., and Pena-Paez, A. (1984). Effects of aging on the recall of extended expository prose. *Exp. Aging Res.*, 10, 25–28.

Till, R. E. (1985). Verbatim and inferential memory in young and elderly adults. *J. Gerontol.*, 40, 316–323.

Toole, T., Pyne, A., and McTarsney, P. A. (1984). Age differences in memory for movements. *Exp. Aging Res.*, 10, 205–210.

Vrtunski, P. B., Patterson, M. B., and Hill, G. O. (1984). Factor analysis of choice reaction time in young and elderly subjects. *Percept. Motor Skill*, 59, 659–676.

Waddell, K. J., and Rogoff, B. (1981). Effect of contextual organization on spatial memory of middle-aged and older women. *Dev. Psychol.*, 17, 878–885.

Walsh, D. A., and Thompson, L. W. (1978). Age differences in visual sensory memory. *J. Gerontol.*, 33, 383–387.

Walsh, D. A., Williams, M. V., and Hertzog, C. K. (1979). Age-related differences in two stages of central perceptual processes: The effects of short duration targets and criterion differences. *J. Gerontol.*, 34, 234–241.

Watkins, M. J. and Watkins, O. C. (1980). The modality effect and echoic persistence. *J. Exp. Psychol.: General*, 109, 251–278.

Welford, A. T. (1985). Changes of performance with age: an overview. In N. Charness (Ed.), *Aging and Human Performance*. New York: John Wiley & Sons, pp. 333–369.

Wingfield, A., Poon, L. W., Lombardi, L., and Lowe, D. (1985). Speed of processing in normal aging: effects of speech rate, linguistic structure, and processing time. *J. Gerontol.*, 40, 579–585.

Wright, L. L., and Elias, J. W. (1979). Age differences in the effects of perceptual noise. *J. Gerontol.*, 34, 704–708.

Wright, R. E. (1981). Aging, divided attention, and processing capacity. *J. Gerontol.*, 36, 605–614.

Yesavage, J. A., and Jacob, R. (1984). Effects of relaxation and mnemonics on memory, attention and anxiety in the elderly. *Exp. Aging Res.*, 10, 211–214.

CHAPTER 9

Input and output

The main problems for the elderly in communicating with their environment derive from the impairment in peripheral systems, i.e. sense organs and locomotor apparatus. These are more important than changes in the central computer, i.e. the brain.

Any information processing system must first have information and in the elderly the transmission of information between the brain and the outside world is frequently impaired.

To begin with the visual input, it is a common experience that the first symptom of aging in a middle-aged man is the need to wear spectacles for reading. Visual threshold for contour detection is defined as the lowest flash intensity at which subjects correctly report the orientation (45° left or right from vertical) of a narrow black line (0.5×65 mm). The age-dependent decrease in detectability is described with accuracy in Fig. 9.1. Intensity is changed by means of neutral filters. The threshold changes with age (df: 10,200; $F = 16.51; p < 0.001$). The values are normally quite steady until age 50, whereafter the function sharply declines.

In white light, only a third of the input flux reaches the retina in the elderly. The sensory visual store suffers a 15% reduction in capacity compared to younger controls, even though that decrease is not considered to be of great importance for subsequent memory stores (Walsh and Thompson, 1978). In fact, when colours

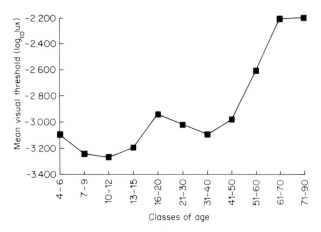

Fig. 9.1   Age and visual threshold for 211 male subjects. Adapted from Dustman et al., 1981, with permission

and sharp contours are tachistoscopically presented to young and elderly subjects (18 msec) no differences are seen (Giaquinto et al., 1985).

In the elderly, the refractive structures of the eye become opaque and the probability of cornea guttata, glaucoma and cataract is increased. The cornea is frail and less sensitive after the 40s. Contact lenses may be harmful, because the subject may be unaware of the damage caused by unsuitable lenses (Millodot and Owens, 1984).

Cataract is present in 9% of the 60–69 age group, but in 36% of subjects over 80 years of age. In this group of people, 36% have 20/50 vision or less in the better eye, and 50% of the subjects have 20/50 vision or less in the other eye (Anderson and Palmore, 1974). These authors also find that the overall probability of an opaque lens rises from 8.2 to 29.8% from 55 to 79 years, irrespective of the sex and eye differences displayed in Table 9.1. However, there are large individual

Table 9.1   Percentages of opaque lens

Classes of age (years)	55–64	65–74	75–79
Men			
Right eye	8.9	10.6	25.9
Left eye	10.3	11.0	22.7
Women			
Right eye	6.6	19.7	33.6
Left eye	7.0	20.4	37.0

differences in these refractive changes in the elderly as we saw in the case of cognitive abilities in the last chapter. As a result the variance is large in responses to stimuli of different spatial frequency, and in particular reaction times may be greatly lengthened, when the spatial frequency goes beyond 6 c/deg and slower visual channels are activated (Kline et al., 1983).

Pupil size decreases from a mean diameter of 4.9 mm in the adolescent to 3.15 mm in the 70–79 age group, bringing about a 0.38 log luminance decrease in retinal illumination. In spite of that correction, both the dark adapted and the scotopic electroretinogram change with age (Wright et al., 1985).

The hard-of-hearing grandfather is a familiar stereotype. Acoustic thresholds increase and 'phonetically balanced words' are less well discriminated (Jerger, 1973). Mean values of audiological threshold in normal subjects are plotted against age (Figs. 9.2 and 9.3). Hearing loss increases with age but only at high

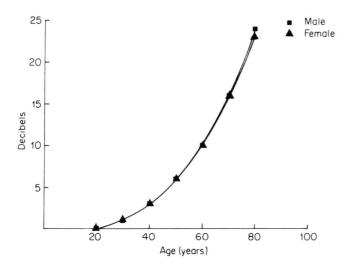

Fig. 9.2   Age-dependent hearing loss. At 1000 Hz there is no-sex difference. Courtesy of Dr. G. C. Passeri

frequencies. This should be carefully checked if it can be done without distressing the subject, who is likely to be ready to quit on account of fatigue or frustration. Hearing loss is mainly due to mechanical factors like the stiffness of the tympanic membrane and in the transmission in the middle ear, or cochlear changes. There is no change with age in the ability to comprehend language when lip-reading or face-reading is available and there is no change as a simple function of age in conditions of high predictability and high signal-to-noise ratio (Obler et al., 1985). However, old subjects are less able than young ones to take

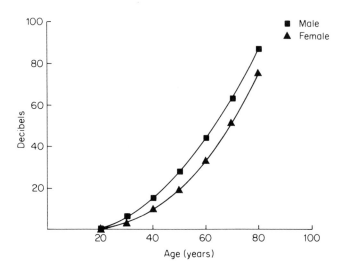

Fig. 9.3   Age-dependent hearing loss. At 8000 Hz women outscore men. Courtesy of Dr. G. C. Passeri

advantage of an improvement in the acoustic environment (Yanz and Anderson, 1984), presumably because of declining high frequency sensitivity.

Saccadic movements are slower in the elderly when localizing a target, but accuracy is not greatly impaired (Warabi et al., 1984). Optokinetic nystagmus performance clearly decreases over the life span. The maximal velocity generally decreases every year by 1°/sec. This is not restricted to ages above 60 but in part of a continuum already identifiable in middle age. Both smooth pursuit and optokinetic afternystagmus velocity decreases with age, these being measures of the fast and the velocity storage components respectively (Simons and Buettner, 1985). It is hard to identify the relative responsibility of peripheral and central mechanisms in these changes. Vestibulo-ocular responses decrease with age. The overall sensitivity of the system is reduced except probably at the highest frequency of sinusoidal stimulation. The response to rotational acceleration stimulation in the oldest subjects is 84.4% compared to younger controls and women have higher average gains than men at the lowest test frequencies (Wall et al., 1984). Unfortunately, in this study the oldest subjects are only 59 years old.

Shakespeare reminds us of the changes in the sensation of taste and odour when Jaques says 'sans taste, sans everything' (see Chapter 1). More recent authors find that the sensitivity to sugar, salt, bitter and acidic substances probably does not decline with age (Byrd and Gertman, 1959; Cohen and Gitman, 1959). The conclusions may seem a little strange, because it is a common experience that the food cooked by grandmother is often too salty, apparently due to her higher threshold. However, odour ability decreases in 80% of subjects over 65 years and this loss will certainly affect tasting. Moreover, taste buds become atrophic with age, the flow of saliva and the ptyalin content are reduced (Ritchie, 1982), thus leading to a peripheral blockage of sensory information. A sex difference has been recognized among the elderly, because women recognize flavours better than men. On the other hand young women outscore old women on olfactory discrimination (Murphy, 1985). The sex difference may depend on the development of particular skills through experience in housework. The better performance of women is supported by experiments using microencapsulated odours (Doty et al., 1984). Average ability reaches a peak between 20 and 40 years and then declines monotonically. A high percentage of elderly people have a major olfactory impairment and may complain about the lack of food flavour. Poor olfactory ability not only affects the enjoyment of day-to-day life, but also it hampers an early warning system for the detection of dangerous fumes, especially fire in the home.

In skeletal muscle the most evident age-related change is the reduction in muscle volume, a fact which might reflect a reduction in either the fibre size or the total number of fibres themselves. In post-mortem material it has been observed that while the size of old muscles is 18% smaller than that of young controls, the total number of fibres is 25% lower. The finding suggests that the reduction in muscle volume typical of the elderly is due to a reduction in the total number of fibers, at least up to the age of 70 (Lexell et al., 1983). Whether the loss of fibres depends on denervation or on small injuries is still undetermined. Type 1 'slow' fibres seem to be better preserved in the aged, whereas type 2, 'fast' fibres suffer a loss of 60%. However, the tendency toward an increase in the slow fibres is not statistically significant. A tendency towards more homogeneous distribution of fibre types is also seen, probably for a slow adaptation reflecting the changes in the physical activity.

Examination of healthy elderly people after vigorous exercise, enough to halve the high energy phosphate reserve and lower the intracellular pH, indicates that the energetics of human skeletal muscle do not change with age (Taylor et al., 1984). The pH variation is similar to that in controls and is consistent with the variation in the phosphocreatine concentration during exercise. Moreover, restitution of phosphocreatine is not affected by the aging process. The observations indicate that both the glycolytic response to muscle contraction and the aerobic capacity for energy synthesis are preserved.

On the other hand, it has been found that both maximum voluntary contraction and supramaximal tetanic contractions are reduced in the elderly. The reduction in voluntary force is greater in the leg muscles than in the arm muscles (McDonagh et al., 1984). The atrophy of muscle fibres with aging obviously affects muscle force. The decrease in fibre number and fibre size, especially for type 2, may be an explanation because it is greater in vastus lateralis than in the biceps brachii (Grimby et al., 1982). As we have seen an alternative explanation is that all fibre types may slow over the life span. Electromyographic findings are in arrangement with the latter hypothesis.

A compilation of the literature on the increase in duration of motor unit potentials with age provides us with data for the muscles of the neck, trunk and limbs (Figs. 9.4, 9.5, 9.6 and 9.7). It is worth noting that muscles involved in

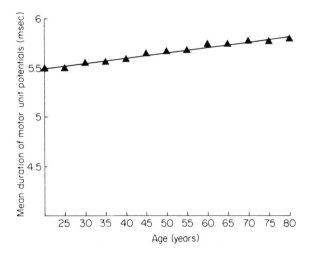

Fig. 9.4   Muscles of the head. Mean duration of motor unit potentials (MUP) as a function of age. Good stability with age. Adapted from data of different sources in the literature, collected and kindly supplied by Dr. A. Rosenfalck

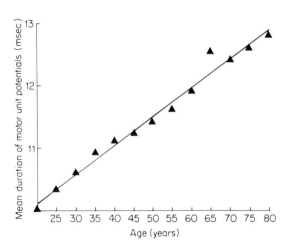

Fig. 9.5   Muscles of the trunk. Linear increase in mean duration of MUP with age

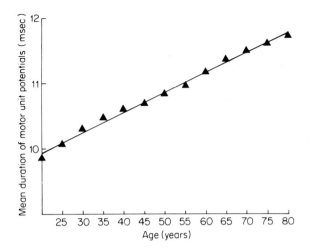

Fig. 9.6   Muscles of the upper limb. Linear increase in the mean duration of MUP with age

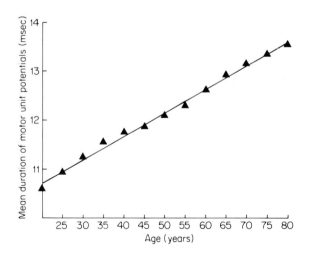

Fig. 9.7   Muscles of the lower limb. Linear increase in the mean duration of MUP with age

respiration and mastication undergo the least modification over the human life span. The chronological order of activation during early infancy is thus reversed in the elderly. The macroelectrode motor unit potential is increased in amplitude perhaps because of reinnervation following clinically silent neural damage (Stalberg and Fawcett, 1982). In this study, the increase in amplitude is particularly evident at the level of the lower limb, a variation which probably explains the increase in the latency of intentional activity (Mankovski et al., 1982).

Under low tension, for instance 20% of maximal contraction, the motor unit discharge has long and irregular interspike intervals with a 'negative floating serial correlation'. In other words, a long interval may follow a short one and vice versa, but intervals are shorter at low tension (Nelson et al., 1984). These authors argue that small motor units are inactive, since the tonic threshold for discharge is not reached and they are therefore replaced by larger motor units. Small and skilled movements at low tension would have a preventive effect in the elderly, especially if they were reinforced by visual feed-back. In many instances the disuse syndrome may be the actual cause of motor problems in this expanding segment of society, more than age itself (Payton and Poland, 1983; Lewis, 1984).

Conduction velocity is reduced with age. It has been calculated that the decrease over the life span is well approximated by a second order polynomial equation. The conduction velocity in the median nerve decreases from 62 to 52 m/sec, albeit not linearly, especially after age 40 (Simpson and Erwin, 1983). Differences in sensory and motor conduction velocities of different nerves are shown in Fig. 9.8. It is worth noting that, contrary to the idea of a maturation

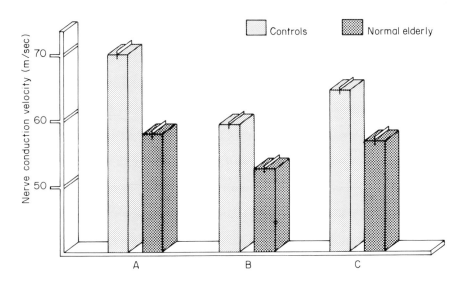

Fig. 9.8 Age-dependent changes in conduction velocity. Y-axis: m/sec. A = musculo-cutaneous nerve. B = median nerve (motor). C = median nerve (sensory)

during adolescence, conduction velocities and amplitude attain their maximum at the fourth decade; from the next decade onwards, sensory and motor conduction velocity and sensory amplitude decline at an increasing rate with a corresponding increase in sensory duration, as measured by the difference between the peak latency and the onset latency of the potentials (Taylor, 1984). The rate of change is the same for both motor and sensory nerves in both upper and lower limbs. The ulnar nerve is an exception, because its sensory amplitude begins to decline as early as the third decade, and these changes bear a linear relationship with age.

With increasing age peripheral nerve endings release less acetylcholine for each action potential, leading to synaptic depression (Smith, 1982). Less diffusion of potassium occurs away from the nerve ending in aged rats than in controls during repetitive stimulation and so there is accumulation of extracellular potassium at the nerve terminal membrane. More terminals and vesicles are found at the endplate of a sprouting process but Smith is unable to confirm that there is an increased acetylcholine content. Recently, mainly acetylcholine receptors have been identified, as small clusters at the endplate and there is an increase in the number of branches of the preterminal axon entering the endplate (Oda, 1984). Fewer endplates are innervated by a single, unbranched preterminal axon. Perijunctional acetylcholine receptors can also be observed in normal aging. They are known to appear either in newborns or disused skeletal fibres, but extrajunctional acetylcholine receptors, i.e. markers of denervation, are never found.

Taken together, these findings seem to indicate true adaptive mechanisms. The hypothesis of a slow and mild denervation–reinnervation process, similar to the enzymatic activities shown in Figs. 5.6 and 5.7, seems to be supported by the finding of increased fibre density and jitter in the elderly (Shields et al., 1984). The mild increase in fibre density, i.e. the number of time-locked single EMG potentials of the same motor unit is correlated with jitter. This finding suggests the formation of new immature neuromuscular junctions with irregular transmission. However, an increased usage of the hand does not increase collateral sprouting and reinnervation nor delay the aging process. On the other hand, the active elderly involved in sport show no decrease in the amplitude of the achilles tendon jerk (deVries et al., 1985). Physical activity may be as important in keeping normal function in the central nervous system as in maintaining muscle structure and function. More data on this topic will be discussed in Chapter 11.

The handgrip task provides a standard motor test of strength. Its average value decreases from 50 kg at age 20 to 36.5 kg at age 70–79. There is a sex difference, but superiority of males fluctuates throughout the life span (Fig. 9.9). Decline of physical performance with time is related to task difficulty, since common tasks decline by 0.5% per year whereas maximal performance declines by 1.5% per year (Stones and Kozma, 1985).

On the tapping task (Fig. 9.10) we observe the expected reduction in score among the elderly (Table 9.2), but we also observe paradoxically that the older group is not very affected by fatigue. The reason seems to be that the elderly employ conservative strategies, avoiding a brisk start, that would bring early exhaustion (Table 9.3).

Another important output, the human voice, undergoes typical age-depen-

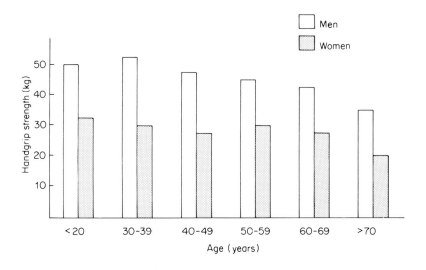

Fig. 9.9   Changes of the handgrip strength with age. Adapted from Stones and Kozma, 1985, with permission

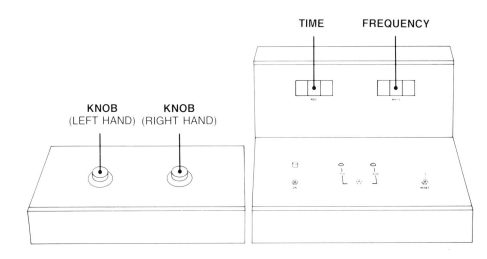

Fig. 9.10   Tapping apparatus. Young subjects outscore normal elderly, but the latter use a conservative strategy and can endure fatigue

Table 9.2 Tapping in right-handed subjects

	N	Mean	S.D.	LCL (.95)	UCL(.95)
Right hand					
Elderly	48	5.23	.78	5.00	5.46
Controls	100	6.41	.94	6.26	6.59
Left hand					
Elderly	48	4.57	.93	4.30	4.84
Controls	100	5.84	.83	4.84	6.00

Table 9.3 Tapping. Decrease in performance after four consecutive trials of 15 sec each. Right-handed subjects

Hand	Elderly	Controls
Right	−11%	−11%
Left	−16.52%	−12.15%

dent changes. Some of them have already been noted, albeit in a poetical form, in the first chapter. Expressive language may be fundamentally altered. Speech may become slow, with few and considered words. The poverty of speech is characterised by an increase in the repetition of words and ideas, anomia with verbal standstill especially for proper nouns, exaggerated gesture, a tendency to use stereotypes and generic words such as 'things' and to leave sentences unfinished (Critchley, 1984).

All movement needs sensory feedback for its successful execution. There is evidence for age related changes in the information from feedback of information to muscles, joints and skin. Studies of the ability to reproduce the perceived position of each knee with the contralateral one and to reproduce return to rest clearly reveal such changes (Kaplan et al., 1985). There is a wide variation both in the threshold values for perceived position changes and in the accuracy in reproducing positions. Nevertheless the authors argue that disability in proprioception and joint position sense may play a more important role in falls and limb fractures in the elderly than changes in the bone itself.

Thresholds for tactile vibration increase with age, especially after the age of 50. The structure of Meissner's corpuscles suggest that they are receptors of mechanical stimuli and their number significantly decreases over the life span. However, the tactile vibration threshold may be increased to the same extent by a reduction in body temperature and by the changes in sensory conduction velocity. The low frequency threshold, measured at 25 Hz, is quite steady with age, but changes have been confirmed for the frequency range 40–250 Hz both in cross-sectional and longitudinal studies (Verrillo and Verrillo, 1985).

It is important to consider the question of pain perception in the elderly. It is generally agreed that an increase in threshold occurs. It has been observed that minor surgery can be performed with minimal anaesthesia in the elderly. Acute coronary occlusions can be asymptomatic, whereas there is a paradoxical increase of subjective complaints (Botwinick, 1984). Data on the cold pressure test indicate that the endorphinic response may be equal or slightly decreased in the elderly compared to younger controls, but it is not increased. This somewhat paradoxical result reminds us that pain perception involves personality traits and affective behaviour as well as objective peripheral mechanisms. In this context it is interesting that elderly people seem particularly sensitive to placebo. In the case of mental stress and postural stimulation plasma norepinephrine (NE) increases in the elderly, compared to young controls (Barnes et al., 1982; Sowers et al., 1983). High plasma NE concentrations in the elderly are due to the rate at which NE enters the circulation, whereas NE production is steady with age (Hoeldtke and Cilmi, 1985).

Summing up, the decline with age of input and output functions is a more important source of impairment than the slowing of central process capabilities, that we have examined in the previous chapter. First of all, the peripheral system transmits information serially. Sensory organs like the eye and ear are examples. In the eye, the cornea, the aqueous humour, the lens, the vitreous body, retina and optic nerve are sequentially traversed by light and the impulses it triggers. Likewise, in the ear, the tympanic membrane, the ossicular chain, oval window, vibrating structures of the cochlea, and the spiral ganglion show a similar serial organization. If only one of these elements is defective, the transmission is affected as a whole, like Christmas tree lights with a defective bulb. Similarly, muscle spindles and other stretch receptors, afferent fibres and the spinal ganglion are serially arranged, and the motor pathway comprises the motoneuron, nerve fibre, endplate, muscle fibre and joint. The chain can be blocked in any of the components and the probability of impaired transmission is related to the length of the chain and the number of the elements involved. For instance, joint position changes in arthritis are also age dependent. Moreover the loss of sensory innervation in the joint can damage the cartilage and worsen the arthritis itself (Skinner et al., 1984), while denervation affects muscle fibres and impairs voluntary force. By contrast, parallel transmission is prevalent in the central nervous system. Here, the probability of saving at least part of the incoming information is higher. For example, recent data on auditory processing of speech indicates that a decline in perception is not age dependent, except in the area of hearing loss (Grady et al., 1984).

Considerations such as these emphasize the greater vulnerability of the peripheral system to age-related deterioration. Ecologically based research, which focuses on both the individual and the environmental situation, is a multivariate approach and is therefore likely to reveal the particular importance of peripheral loss in everyday competence.

There is one more reason for the major role of peripheral defects in the declining interaction of the elderly with his environment. Plasticity and restorative mechanisms in the central nervous system are more likely to effect at least a partial recovery. After a stroke some degree of movement often returns, in spite of the loss of cortical and subcortical areas. By contrast, cataract and ankylosis cannot change for the better in an old person, even though his brain is as fresh as a teenager's. It follows that a cognitively bright elderly person, who can master the hardest professional problems, may have difficulty in reading or going upstairs. His life is increasingly disadvantaged and under the burden of his peripheral problems he shows a progressive loss of interest, voluntary confinement at home and increased introspection. Depression is on the doorstep.

REFERENCES

Anderson, B., and Palmore, E. (1974). Longitudinal evaluation of ocular function. In E. Palmore (Ed.), *Normal Aging. II.* Durham, N. C.: The Duke University Press, pp. 115–126.

Barnes, R. F., Raskind, M., Gumbrecht, G., and Halter, J. B. (1982). The effect of age on the plasma catecholamine response to mental stress in man. *J. Clin. Endocrinol. Metab.*, 54, 64–69.

Botwinick, J. (1984). *Aging and Behaviour.* New York: Springer Publ. Co.

Byrd, E., and Gertman, S. (1959). Taste sensitivity in aged persons. *Geriatrics*, 14, 381–384.

Cohen, T., and Gitman, I. (1959). Oral complaints and taste perception in the aged. *J. Gerontol.*, 14, 294–298.

Critchley, M. (1984). And all the daughters of musick shall be brought low. Language function in the elderly. *Arch. Neurol.*, 41, 1135–1139.

deVries, H. A., Wiswell, R. A., Romero, G. T., and Heckathorne, E. (1985). Changes with age in monosynaptic reflexes elicited by mechanical and electrical stimulation. *Amer. J. Phys. Med.*, 64, 71–81.

Doty, R. L., Shaman, P., Applebaum, S. L., Giberson, R., Siksorski, L., and Rosenberg, L. (1984). Smell identification ability: changes with age. *Science*, 226, 1441–1443.

Dustman, R. E., Snyder, R. W., and Schlehuber, C. J. (1981). Life-span alterations in visually evoked potentials and inhibitory functions. *Neurobiol. Aging*, 2, 187–192.

Giaquinto, S., Nolfe, G., and Calvani, M. (1985). Cluster analysis of cognitive performance in elderly and demented subjects. *Ital. J. Neurol. Sci.*, 6, 157–165.

Grady, C. L., Grimes, A. M., Pikus, A., Schwartz, M., Rapoport, S. I., and Cutler, N. R. (1984). Alterations in auditory processing of speech stimuli during aging in healthy subjects. *Cortex*, 20, 101–110.

Grimby, G., Danneskiold-Samsøe, B., Hoid, K., and Saltin, B. (1982). Morphology and enzymatic capacity in arm and leg muscles in 78–81 year old men and women. *Acta Physiol. Scand.*, 115, 125–134.

Hoeldtke, R. D., and Cilmi, K. M. (1985). Effects of aging on catecholamine metabolism. *J. Clin. Endocrinol. Metab.*, 60, 479–484.

Jerger, J. (1973). Audiological findings in aging. *Adv. Otorhynolaring.*, 20, 115–124.

Kaplan, F. S., Nixon, J. E., Reitz, M., Rindfleish, L., and Tucker, J. (1985). Age-related change in proprioception and sensation of joint position. *Acta Orthop. Scand.*, 56, 72–74.

Kline, D. W., Schieber, F., Abusamra, L. C., and Coyne, A. C. (1983). Age, the eye and the visual channels: contrast sensitivity and response speed. *J. Gerontol.*, 38, 211–216.

Lewis, C. B. (1984). Rehabilitation of the older person: a psychosocial focus. *Phys. Ther.*, 64, 517–522.

Lexell, J., Henriksson-Larsén, K., Winblad, B., and Sjøstrøm, M. (1983). Distribution of different fiber types in human skeletal muscles: effects of aging studied in whole muscle cross sections. *Muscle & Nerve*, 6, 588–595.

Mankovski, N. B., Mints, A. Y., and Lisenyuk, V. P. (1982). Age peculiarities of human motor control in aging. *Gerontology*, 28, 314–322.

McDonagh, M. J. N., White, M. J., and Davies, C. T. M. (1984). Different effects of ageing on the mechanical properties of human arm and leg muscles. *Gerontology*, 30, 49–54.

Millodot, M., and Owens, H. (1984). The influence of age on the fragility of cornea. *Acta ophthalmol.*, 62, 819–824.

Murphy, C. (1985). Cognitive and chemosensory influences on age-related changes in the ability to identify blended foods. *J. Gerontol.*, 40, 47–52.

Nelson, R. M., Soderberg, G. L., and Urbscheit, N. L. (1984). Alteration of motor-unit discharge characteristics in aged humans. *Phys. Ther.*, 64, 29–34.

Obler, L. K., Nicholas, M., Albert, M. L., and Woodward, S. (1985). On comprehension across the adult lifespan. *Cortex*, 21, 273–280.

Oda, K. (1984). Age changes of motor innervation and acetylcholine receptor distribution on human skeletal muscle fibres. *J. Neurol. Sci.*, 66, 327–338.

Payton, O. D., and Poland, J. L. (1983). Aging process. Implications for clinical practice. *Phys. Ther.*, 63, 41–48.

Ritchie, J. M. (1982). Some pathophysiological aspects of neuronal aging, In R. D. Terry, C. L. Bolis and G. Toffano (Eds), *Aging*, vol. 18. New York: Raven Press, pp. 89–98.

Shields, R. W., Robbins, N., and Verrilli, A. A. (1984). The effects of chronic muscular activity on age-related changes in single fiber electromyography. *Muscle & Nerve*, 7, 273–277.

Simons, B., and Buettner, U. (1985). The influence of age on optokinetic nystagmus. *Eur. Arch. Psychiatr. Neurol. Sci.*, 234, 369–373.

Simpson, D. M., and Erwin, C. W. (1983). Evoked potential latency change with age suggests differential aging of primary somatosensory cortex. *Neurobiol. of Aging*, 4, 59–63.

Skinner, H. B., Barrack, R. L., and Cook, S. D. (1984). Age-related decline in proprioception. *Clin. Orthop.*, 184, 208–211.

Smith, D. O. (1982). Physiological and structural changes at the neuromuscular junction during aging. In E. Giacobini, G. Filogamo, G. Giacobini and A. Vernadakis (Eds), *Aging*, vol. 20. New York: Raven Press, pp. 123–137.

Sowers, J. R., Rubenstein, L. Z., and Stern, N. (1983). Plasma norepinephrine response to posture and isometric exercise increase with age in the absence of obesity. *J. Gerontol.*, 38, 315–317.

Stalberg, E., and Fawcett, P. R. (1982). Macro EMG in healthy subjects of different ages. *J. Neurol. Neurosurg. Psychiat.*, 45, 870–878.

Stones, M. J., and Kozma, A. (1985). Physical performance. In Charness N. (Ed.), *Aging and Human Performance*. New York: John Wiley & Sons, pp. 261–291.

Taylor, P. K. (1984). Non-linear effects of age on nerve conduction in adults. *J. Neurol. Sci.*, 66, 223–234.

Taylor, D. J., Crowe, M., Bore, P. J., Styles, P., Arnold, D. L., and Radda, G. K. (1984). Examination of the energetics of aging skeletal muscle using nuclear magnetic resonance. *Gerontology*, 30, 2–7.

Verrillo, R. T., and Verrillo, V. (1985). Sensory and perceptual performance. In Charness N. (Ed.), *Aging and Human Performance*. New York: John Wiley & Sons, pp. 1–46.

Wall III, C., Black, F. O., and Hunt, A. E. (1984). Effect of age, sex and stimulus parameters upon vestibulo-ocular responses to sinusoidal rotation. *Acta Otolaryngol. (Stock.)*, 98, 270–278.

Walsh, D. A., Williams, M. V., and Hertzog, C. K. (1979). Age-related differences in two stages of central perceptual processes: The effects of short duration targets and criterion differences. *J. Gerontol.*, 34, 234–241.

Warabi, T., Kase, M., and Kato, T. (1984). Effect of aging on the accuracy of visually guided saccadic eye movement. *Ann. Neurol.*, 16, 449–454.

Wright, C. E., Williams, D. E., Drasdo, N., and Harding, G. F. A. (1985). The influence of age on the electroretinogram and visual evoked potential. *Doc. Ophthalmol.*, 59, 365–384.

Yanz, Y. L., and Anderson, S. M. (1984). Comparison of speech perception skills in young and old listeners. *Ear Hear*, 5, 64–71.

CHAPTER 10

Illnesses of the older brain

The sociological literature often places the aged in a single category, as if they were all alike. Accurate diagnoses permit us to intervene purposefully, often with positive results.

Although this book is mainly concerned with the normal elderly, it is appropriate to list the main neurological and psychiatric disturbances which commonly affect them. The hypothesis of a causal connection between advanced age and frequent illness is unlikely to be correct, as we have already seen. The increased incidence of ill health in this group may have an indirect cause in the risk factors connected with age, which we discussed in relation to the cerebral blood flow. Some disorders which seem more common in the elderly may be due to slow neuropathological processes which begin in youth or middle age and only reveal themselves in individuals who happen to survive long enough. Indeed, studies of cerebral flow, metabolism, neurophysiology and neuropsychology all tell us that gradual changes take place in the nervous system after the 30s. In part, these changes are detectable, but in part they are masked by strategies of adaptation and recovery.
    The typical diseases of old age are the following:

1) Alzheimer's disease (AD/SD or SDAT)
2) Multi-infarct dementia (MID)
3) Mixed dementia

4) Pick's dementia
5) Binswanger's subcortical encephalopathy
6) Parkinson's disease
7) Hyperkinesias of various origins
8) Idiopathic hydrocephalus
9) Progressive supranuclear palsy (PSP)
10) Creutzfeld–Jakob's disease
11) Depression
12) Neurosis
13) Psychosis and confusional states

We shall look at each of these disorders in turn.

ALZHEIMER'S DEMENTIA

The Diagnostic and Statistical Manual of Mental Disorders says that senile dementia is a syndrome including progressive mental deterioration, loss of memory and cognitive functions with resulting inability to carry out daily activities. The illness affects older individuals, but it also strikes younger subjects in good physical health and in this case it is called pre-senile dementia. This terminology has been criticized, however, because it suggests that there is a dementia caused by old age (Liston, 1979).

The Anglo-Saxon tendency to use acronyms has now produced the term AD/SD (Alzheimer's disease/senile dementia), which unifies these pathologies. The term SDAT (senile dementia of Alzheimer's type) is also used. AD/SD refers to a primary dementia. From histological studies of the basal nucleus of Meynert (see Chapter 4), it seems that AD should be distinguished from SD, because in the latter form the basal nucleus is spared and the clinical pattern is different. There are further arguments for distinguishing the two forms, based on the finding of differences in the concentration of neurotransmitters and enzymatic activities in AD and SD (Gottfries, 1985). The clinical patterns and progression of these disorders are also different. The AD group is more homogeneous with a marked wasting pathology, while the clinical pathology of the senile group is slower and more easily confused with the natural involution of more advanced age. AD mainly affects semantic processing (agnosia, apraxia and aphasia), while SD mainly affects memory. At the same time, epidemiological studies suggest that Alzheimer's dementia should not be divided into pre-senile and senile forms based only on the time of onset, because the expected bimodal distribution curve is not found (Rocca et al., 1986). The incidence of AD/SD varies greatly among the different reports (Pinessi et al., 1984; Rocca et al., 1986; Khachaturian, 1985). In any event the statistical data indicate that the disorder will affect an increasing proportion of the population in the future, with age an important risk factor (Fig. 10.1).

The cause or causes have not yet been identified. Epidemiological studies so far indicate that the majority of cases are sporadic. Nevertheless there are a

Table 10.1   Hachinski's ischaemic score

Score	Symptom
2 points	Abrupt onset Fluctuation History of stroke Focal symptoms Focal signs
1 point	Stepwise deterioration Nocturnal confusion Relative preservation of personality Depression Somatic complaints Emotional lability Hypertension Other signs of arteriosclerosis

A score of 4 or less points to AD/SD.
A score of 6 or more points to MID.

version achieves even better results (Table 10.2). In the case of MID, the differential diagnosis must also take into account tumours, alcoholism, cranial traumas, metabolic disturbances and drug effects.

Simple arteriosclerosis does not cause dementia unless it also causes organic lesions. They can take the form of a single large infarct, or multiple infarcts of medium size, or alterations of the white matter, such as a perivascular fibrinolytic activity (Tohgi, 1985). From the tables it is evident that vascular disorders have the major role in determining both the onset and the course of the illness. The focal neurological signs can be diverse, including motor, phasic, sensorial, mnesic disturbances and the symptoms may include paraesthesias, pain and general disperceptive phenomena. The step-wise deterioration is more clearly marked in MID than in AD/SD, because there is generally a clinical interval between one cerebrovascular episode and another which becomes shorter and shorter. It has recently been suggested that AD/SD can be distinguished from MID because on tests of learning and memory, the use of visuospatial cues for recall is more strongly affected than the rote learning of auditory verbal material (Muramoto, 1984). The observation points to a primary impairment of the right hemisphere in AD/SD. However, it is important to note that the author has probably biased the results of this study by excluding aphasic disturbances and that the comparison of different pathological groups introduces problems of uniformity. Very often, MID is recognized on the occasion of a new and more evident cerebral vascular illness. The CT scan shows former multiple foci in addition to the recent lesion and the history reveals the signs of deterioration which are accentuated after the new episode. In the case of vascular diseases, there may also be epileptic seizures, but these are without any characteristics peculiar to the aged (Haan, 1983). It has been calculated that the prevention of the major causes of death, represented by

Table 10.2   Modified ischaemic score

Symptom	Score
Abrupt onset	2
History of stroke	1
Focal symptoms	2
Focal signs	2
CT: Low density areas	
isolated	2
multiple	3
Multiple Score =	10

(from Loeb and Gandolfo, 1983)

cardiovascular diseases, would increase life expectancy by 10 years (Katzman, 1983). Patients who do survive longer as a result of improvements in the treatment of, for example, coronary heart disease will greatly enlarge the risk group for MID.

MIXED FORMS OF DEMENTIA

In spite of Hachinski's scale, differentiation can be difficult in some cases. Apart from this scale even Alzheimer's dementia is diagnosed on the basis of simple exclusion. Sometimes the occurrence of characteristics of more than one type of dementia does not allow a clear-cut separation. In spite of the means at our disposal misdiagnosis must be quite frequent. Autopsy evidence for mixed forms accounts for 18% of cases (Tomlinson et al., 1970). Mixed forms have been separately classified and perhaps represent one of the many examples in medicine where the thinking is not clearly stated. Nuclear Magnetic Resonance is very useful for the proper diagnosis of AD/SD patients, because if they have small infarcts in the white matter the AD/SD diagnosis is unlikely.

A brain biopsy would clear up any diagnostic doubts, but ethical, political and practical considerations render this technique very rare as a diagnostic procedure. In fact it is important that we clarify the neurochemical and structural changes *in vivo* in order to advance the basic knowledge of these wasting and still incurable diseases. The histological and histochemical observations of a small fragment of non-cadaveric neural tissue could one day give us the key that not even PET has given us.

PICK'S DEMENTIA

This condition is similar in many respects to AD/SD but it selectively affects only the frontal and the temporal lobes, sparing the posterior part of the temporal gyri, as well as the occipital lobes. Pick's dementia is rare and has a more precocious onset than classical AD/SD. It generally begins before 65 years of age, although the original case described by Pick was 71 years old (Alexander and Geschwind,

1984). Frontal signs prevail with initial alterations of temper, apathy, foolish behaviour and tendency towards infantile banter. The course of the disease is more or less like that of AD/SD, 2 to 10 years after the beginning of the symptoms. Many authors hold that it is not possible to distinguish between the clinical signs of Pick's disease and AD/SD, but there is a substantial body of opinion that personality disturbances and cognitive disorders take priority in Pick's disease. The disturbance consists of emotional blunting, apathy, delirium, irritability, inappropriate social behaviour, echolalia, word searching, verbal stereotypes and alexia. On the other hand memory, visual and spatial functions and motor patterns remain relatively preserved until the disease is well advanced, when bilateral extrapyramidal signs predominate (Alexander and Geschwind, 1984). Two items of information are needed for a definite diagnosis of Pick's dementia. Well-circumscribed atrophy in frontal and temporal regions are seen in the CT scan and a normal EEG. It is interesting that the EEG can be normal in Pick's dementia, while it is not in AD/SD (Gordon and Sim, 1967; Johannesson et al., 1979). For unclear reasons, the diagnosis of Pick's dementia is rare in the USA (Boller et al., 1984).

BINSWANGER'S SUBCORTICAL ENCEPHALOPATHY

This condition is not characterized by a typical clinical picture. The diagnosis is not possible without the aid of the CT scan, or better still by NMR, which shows lesions in the white matter, especially around the frontal horn and in the centrum ovale. Internal hydrocephalus may also be present. It is still unclear whether or not this condition should be considered as a separate disease. According to recent interpretations it may be due to lipohyalinosis and therefore to lacunar infarcts and ischaemic leucoencephalopathy, while MID would be the consequence of a lesion in the larger vessels (Roman, 1985) or systemic lesions without hypertension, or haemorrhages as in the Japanese population (Tohgi, 1985). Clinically, we find pyramidal, extrapyramidal and pseudo-bulbar signs and automatism. Tactile sensitivity and sphincter control do not appear to be impaired.

PARKINSON'S DISEASE

This well-known neurological disease typically occurs in the aged. Nearly non-existent before 40 years of age, 10% of the cases begins in the fifth decade. The highest incidence, amost 40%, occurs between 60 and 70 years of age. Men show the signs slightly earlier than women. The disease affects about 1:1000 of the population, but 1% of people in their 70s. The diagnosis is generally easy because of the characteristic signs. There may be some doubt in the initial phase, especially if the illness begins with infrequent signs. In the great majority of cases, more than two out of three, the tremor is the typical sign, stable at 4–6 Hz, traditionally compared to the act of pill rolling. On the other hand, in 10% of the cases the disease begins with rigidity, which can be unilateral or bilateral, like the tremor. The stiffness is typically plastic, waxy, with cog-wheel rigidity and, in the advanced phase like a lead-pipe. In the younger subjects it usually begins with tremor, while in the older subject the first indication is usually bradykinesia.

Less frequent signs are disturbances of gait, typically in small steps, muscle pain, loss of pendular movement, writing difficulties, loss of dexterity, bradylalia and depression (Dupont, 1980).

In the period of pronounced symptoms, we also observe non-neurological signs, such as seborrhoea, prevalent in males, which is correlated with the seriousness of the clinical pattern and sensitive to the L-DOPA treatment (Baas and Fisher, 1985). Important joint defects occur which can cause disabling deformities in untreated patients. The frequent depression in parkinsonian patients is not correlated with extrapyramidal signs, and therefore seems to be an independent disturbance (Hietanen and Teravainen, 1985). It can recede or remain with treatment for the motor disturbance.

Parkinson's disease may be regarded as a primitive disorder. It constitutes a well-known clinical model of neurochemical deficit. There is a reduction in dopaminergic activity of the nigro-striatal system with a reduction in receptors for dopamine, GABA, acetylcholine and enkephalin (e.g. Gottfries et al., 1980). There is not only degeneration of neurons in the substantia nigra and changes in the D-2 striatal receptors, but there may also be a loss of nigro-striatal neurons as a result of reduced D-1 receptor binding (Rinne et al., 1985).

Secondary parkinsonism is observed in the encephalitic form (even though the surviving cases of the 1917 pandemic are today very few), in cases improperly treated with neuroleptics or flunarizine, and in conditions associated with repeated head injuries as occurs in boxing. A significant percentage of cases, 8%, are of arteriosclerotic origin (Agnoli et al., 1980). The drugs most widely used today in the therapy of Parkinson's disease are anti-cholinergics, amantadine, bromocriptine, lisuride and the widely used L-DOPA. The last provided a real revolution in therapy at the beginning of the 70s but it can accentuate the tremor as well as the dyskinesias and cause on-off phenomena in long-term treatment. For this reason we try to reduce the dosage, resorting to dopaminergic agonists (Stern, 1980; Giovannini, et al., 1983). The L-DOPA itself is always given with an inhibitor, carbidopa or benserazide, in order to block its peripheral effects and concentrate its activity in the brain. Treatment more easily causes dyskinesias in younger patients and hallucinations in older subjects. About 30% of the patients suffering from Parkinson's disease show mental deterioration. These changes are explained by a secondary cholinergic deficit in cortical and subcortical regions and by a decrease in somatostatin levels (Agid et al., 1985; Soininen et al., 1985).

OTHER HYPERKINESIAS

Tremor in the elderly is not always due to Parkinson's disease. In a recent study we observed cases of senile tremor which correspond with familiar tremor (Francolini et al., 1985). Familiar tremor is very different from that of Parkinson's disease, both in frequency and in its appearance during movement and not at rest. This type of tremor, which for simplicity we will refer to as 'essential', affects the upper limbs in two out of three of the cases. Generally, it is evidenced by outstretched arms. In the aged the essential tremor is from 10 to 16 times more common than that of Parkinsons's disease. By contrast, at 40 years of age essential tremor is 140 times more common. It also differs from parkinsonism in that it may occur in adolescence (Dupont, 1980). Partial benefits are achieved with the use of trazodone, anticholinergic drugs and propranolol. Alcohol temporarily dampens the tremor. Other hyperkinesias which may occur in the aged include the familiar degenerative condition of Huntington's disease, and the sporadic so-called senile chorea. The former is associated with serious dementia. Both are characterized by bizarre impulsive movements, accompanied by grimaces. Sometimes the hyperkinesias localize in the mouth–tongue apparatus, the movements being frequent and annoying. They respond to tiapride and pimozide therapy.

IDIOPATHIC HYDROCEPHALUS

The clinical pattern may be indistinguishable from other foms of dementia, but one must be cautious if disturbances of the gait and urinary incontinence precede psychic symptoms. These consist of disturbances of attention, memory, intelligence (in the wider sense) with involvement of the emotional and affective sphere. A history of former brain illnesses is of great significance. It is very important to diagnose this condition because many cases respond to treatment. A professor who was demented and coprophagic, returned to teach at his faculty of agriculture after a ventricular drainage (Guidetti and Gagliardi, 1980). A CT scan is important but not decisive. The finding of hydrocephalus with scarce signs of atrophy on the surface is an important indication. Radioisotope scanning of the cisternae displays the early accumulation of radioiodinate human albumin in the ventricular cavities and none on the cortical spaces even after 48–72 hours. The accumulation can last three days, but even this is not decisive for the diagnosis. Measurement of the intracranial pressure gives the most reliable results, especially if taken directly from the ventricles. After insertion of the shunt, cerebral blood flow and neurological conditions improve over the course of a few months, but mental functions are slower to recover (Meyer et al., 1985; Jørg and Schneider, 1985).

PROGRESSIVE SUPRANUCLEAR PALSY

This illness has the same onset as AD/SD with similar initial symptoms. Slight mental alterations, such as irritability, distrust, and negligence. Later on, there are disturbances of vision and gait with frequent falls, dysarthria and dysphagia. Diagnosis usually comes when the typical supranuclear ophthalmology establishes itself at the beginning, limited to vertical eye movements. The expression is motionless. Speech slows down until anarthria is reached. Dysphagia is particularly dangerous because of the resulting bronchopneumonia *ab ingestis*. The body takes on the posture of hyperextension. There is no treatment for this progressively fatal condition.

CREUTZFELD–JAKOB SYNDROME

This dreadful disease may present itself as early as in the 40s. The characteristics are those of a slow virus infection: a long incubation, but then an inexorable progression and death within a year. The classical signs of the illness include pyramidal and associated extrapyramidal signs, progressive mental decline and myoclonus. Diagnosis is facilitated by the presence of typical EEG complexes, which consist of slow, high voltage, pseudo-periodical paroxysms. The illness begins in an insidious manner with emotional and behavioural disturbances, amnesia, headache, confusion, vertigo and dizziness. Its fast course, the clinical data and the characteristic EEG generally lead to the correct diagnosis, but the neuropathological findings may present variations from case to case (Lechi et al., 1983). The agent is present in other tissues beside the brain and can be transmitted to monkeys by the inoculation of material taken from lymphonodes (Fieschi et al., 1983). There is no cure.

DEPRESSION

Senescence is called the age of loss: loss of work, social status, mate, health, habits, house and sometimes also children (Nakamura, 1982). It is not surprising that many of the aged, spared from dementing illnesses, are caught by depression. Though very different from dementia in biological and psychopathological terms, depression has an effect on cognitive processes, which is sometimes even worse than that of aging itself (Mormont, 1984). A pattern may appear which is incorrectly called 'pseudo-dementia', an ambiguous term which reveals only a diagnostic error from the beginning (Boller et al., 1984; Wertheimer, 1984). Cognitive functions, particularly attention and memory, have not deteriorated, they are simply unexercised. In cases of so-called pseudo-dementia the onset is very swift and affective changes precede cognitive disturbances. The patient may refuse to speak, a fact which emphasizes his disturbance. His performance on neuropsychological tests is unpredictable, variable and unrelated to task difficulty (Wells, 1982). Differential diagnosis is very important, because the depression can be cured with drugs in a relatively short time. By contrast, the diagnosis of dementia may consign the patient to an unsuitable institution, which may in turn accentuate the depression and bring about suicide. The differential diagnosis is made easier by recording the P3 response. Its latency in particular is important (Chapter 7). This, in conjunction with the Mini Mental Scale (Folstein et al., 1975), discriminates those who are only apparently demented. Interest in gerontological research has led to the introduction of a new task battery for depression which is easy to administer. The Geriatric Depression Scale (GDS) consists of the 30 questions best correlated with the final score from an initial set of 100

(Yesavage et al., 1983). This battery classifies subjects into normal and depressed and measures the seriousness of the condition, with sensitivity and specificity.

Description of cognitive function is therefore not always synonymous with organic damage. From a clinical point of view, congruent and mutual variations of cognition, behaviour and effect, would mutually suggest an organic process. This form of depression is clearly an exception, as is schizophrenia where the cognitive changes led the early psychiatrists to refer to it as 'dementia praecox'.

The incidence of depression is high even in the general population. It was identified in 5.4% of a random sample of about 500 citizens in Edinburgh (Williamson, 1980). The diagnosis of depression in the aged may slip by, as it can be masked by hypochondriacal symptoms. These lead the patient to a general physician and are interpreted as signs of a chronic organic illness. Primary depression interferes with vital functions and inhibition can be so marked as to render the patient completely mute, though his gaze reveals sorrow. Appetite and sleep are the first functions to be affected. Sometimes there is concomitant agitation which has the effect of accentuating the depression. The use of neuroleptics may worsen the clinical condition. A feeling of ruin is often the only ideational theme, frequently supported by arguments which appear logically unquestionable. For example, an elderly depressed patient denied the existence of death, affirming that death, funerals and graves were all a pretence. Had her doctor ever exhumed a coffin to verify its contents? Depression in the elderly patient may occur without melancholia, especially in cases formerly affected by stroke and now detached from the outside world. These patients let themselves slowly die without any interest in life. Depression can also be the herald of serious physical illnesses, such as tumour of the pancreas.

Depression may be primed by sudden changes of life style, such as retirement. The elderly person justifies his mood, revealing in particular an anxiety about organizational matters, which appear trivial to an observer but which signal to the patient his inability to cope with the simplest situations.

Depression may be induced in the aged by the excessive use of hypotensive drugs, like alpha-methyl-DOPA, clonidine, the propranolol for their anti-catecholamine effect and reserpine for its anti-serotonin effect. Lastly, the benzodiazepines also accentuate depression in the elderly, further reducing motivational drive.

Just as drugs can cause depression, so they can be responsible for its relief. Response to treatment is excellent in many cases, giving the patient and his family the impression of a recovery that was beyond their hopes and expectations. The anti-MAO are difficult to use in the elderly because they have adverse effects on the circulation and impose severe restrictions on the diet. The side-effects of anti-depressant drugs with anti-cholinergic action (such as tachycardia, dry mouth, drowsiness and asthenia) and their risky use in other illnesses (such as glaucoma and cardiopathy) are largely overcome by the use of so-called second generation antidepressants. No one drug is perfect for all patients. However, they offer the advantage of a rapid action and they are well tolerated by elderly patients (Busse and Simpson, 1983). General measures such as a supportive family environment cannot be totally replaced by drugs. Instead, drugs are to be used only when those measures have not solved the problem. The older patient must continue with the antidepressant treatment, even after it has provided relief because relapses are likely and these are sometimes not reported by the patient (Williamson, 1980).

NEUROSIS

There are two basic questions to be asked about psychopathological changes in the elderly: a) to what extent are they caused by aging itself? b) to what extent are they organic and to what extent 'functional'? These questions are often diffcult to answer in individual cases. Often the diagnosis of a functional disturbance such as neurosis is subject to revision with the use of more sophisticated tests and investigations. In general, it is difficult to accept the idea of a neurotic condition beginning at an advanced age, for this contradicts every psychoanalytic theory. The study of the basic personality, the faithful reconstruction of psychological profile, the recall of episodes in infancy and adolescence, which provide the seeds for neurosis, are very difficult. Moreover, transformation, re-elaboration and cancellation affect memory in the aged (see Chapter 8).

The following classification of neurosis is proposed to cover all neurotic conditions (Gurian and Auerbach, 1984): a) anxiety neurosis, b) depressive neurosis, c) a mixture of anxiety and depressive neurosis, d) hypochondriasis. Similar schemes exist for other disorders. Yet it is often difficult to differentiate the majority of depressions into primary and reactive (Williamson, 1980), except for extreme cases in large populations where the essential patterns can be recognized. In practice, real physical changes, daily variations, sleep disturbances, and dietary upset interfere with the mood and so obscure categorical diagnosis. An understanding of character and the situational disturbances of old age is considered a more valid approach (Gurian and Auerbach, 1984), precisely because it does not attempt an aetiopathogenetic identification, but rather lends itself to individual description. Indeed it is impossible to imagine that a simple classification, such as the DSM-III, can cover all the psychogeriatric disturbances which occur in the USA as well as in Europe, in the north as well as in the south, among professionals and illiterates of different habits, races and cultures. We believe that such classification artificially compartmentalizes psychopathology when, more than ever, there is a complex interplay of factors including the 'organic' and 'functional', somatic and psychic, cognitive and affective.

Many neurotic conditions may even become attenuated in the aged. Phobic and compulsive disorders as well as conversion hysteria become less severe due to the weakening of the ideo-affective complexes, which in these patients would require psychic energy. The same free anxiety may lessen in a subject with a progressive reduction in dopaminergic activity. In the psychopathological phenomena of the aged there is a greater localization of somatic anxiety, with a sharp reduction of exchange with the outside world and a greater need of reassurance and assistance. When it occcurs in advanced age, neurosis is often characterized by a somatic condition. All general physicians known the difficulty in freeing the subject from the bother of his dysfunctions, often varied, concomitant and painful.

Digestive disturbances are very frequent, perhaps even the most frequent of all somatic complaints. Intestinal functions become particularly important and constipation comes to occupy a privileged place in the medical interview, with minute description and continual requests for laxatives. For these reasons the aged show a good knowledge of emulsions, herbal teas and mucilages. In hospital, there is a pressing request for enemas, which provide a real gratification, probably due to regressive phenomena of libido. The wish is so strong, that frequently the patient deliberately lies, reporting a long period of constipation, which is not confirmed by the nurses. Following in frequency, there are musculo-osteo-articular disturbances, where it is often difficult to identify whether the problem is due to fibrosis, or to arthritic or osteoporotic transformations. The diagnosis is often reached by '*ex adjuvantibus*' criteria. A neurotic disturbance which certainly belongs to advanced age is the modification of the conjugal relationship, due to the regressive features in the patient's personality. Though not demented, he treats his wife as a mother and he is pleased to be treated as a baby. Incidentally, in Italian a vernacular synonym for being demented is 'rimbambito', which literally means 'to become a baby again'. I have often heard the elderly patient calling his wife 'Mummy' and she, in turn, appears to be pleased about it. This variation in the relationship is made easier by the waning of the libido, which in turn cancels the unconscious hostility of the mate who is still vigorous.

Regressive elements, such as aggressiveness, hostility, competitiveness and hegemony, are found in elderly people who live in uncongenial surroundings. The Ptolemaic vision of his own ego accentuates the little defeats of a daily life made up of sacrifices, competitions, priorities and monotonous habits. The scarcity of outside stimuli accentuates the lack of self-realization. Injurious behaviour is not infrequent, since the thresholds for spitefulness and irritability are low. The snoring room-mate, or one who is obliged to get up at night to empty his bladder, represents an annoying intrusion on a world characterized by the early awakenings of the elderly.

For the reasons we considered earlier, therapy for these disturbances is not easy. The benzodiazepines are not advised, as they may create confusional states in the elderly. The drugs of choice in this type of geriatric psychopathology are trazodone and L-tryptophan, especially if fast action is not desired.

PSYCHOSIS

Natural aging never causes psychosis. Manic states lessen and catatonic schizophrenic forms are non-existent. It has been said that schizophrenia burns out in old age (Gurian and Auerbach, 1984). When psychotic symptoms do arise, it is often impossible to distinguish organic and 'psychic' factors.

Delusions certainly develop as a result of impairment in communication between the subject and his environment. The reduction of sensory input, the sensitivity to muscular fatigue, the shortening of his own range of action, the difficulty in organizing and directing his thoughts and the effort needed for memory, all make the subject feel a sense of inferiority, from which derive insecurity and a sense of threat.

Loneliness and alienation are not tautological concepts (Wertheimer, 1984), and both may feed mechanisms of projection, making the patient distrustful. Very often, the delusion of persecution is a psychotic defence against frustration. Personal objects put in unusual places, so that they cannot be found, give the patient the idea of theft and attacks on his personal patrimony. Delusions in the elderly patient have structural characteristics, which are fragmentary, scarce and limited to his immediate environment. The patient is distractable and may get better by improving his relationship with the outside world. The term 'paraphrenia' indicates a psychosis of late onset, with bizarre thinking and isolated hallucinations. This type of pathology is not included in DSM-III. Erotomania may be considered a type of 'paraphrenia', like the *Liebewahn* of the German authors, which was firstly described by de Clerambault in the 'excited excitables'. In this form an intense affective polarization drives the subject. As Freud has already pointed out, the formula of erotomania is not derived from passion as it may seem ('I love and I am loved in return'), but rather from unconscious hate. Feelings generating the idea 'I am loved' appear to be pride, desire and hope. Subsequent phases are spitefulness and hate. The subject's conversation with the object is configured into a mental automatism. The continuous presence of the object, the physical influence of the desire of the object, the cohabitation and erotic possession are some elements which induce 'indirect conversations'. Erotomania, which is also considered as a late form of schizophrenia, has probably an organic component stemming from mnemonic and visual-perceptive changes (Lesser et al., 1985).

CONFUSIONAL STATES

The causes of stupor, confusion and/or agitation frequently have a metabolic origin in the aged. The psychiatric disturbances of the aged must always be considered as potentially having metabolic or iatrogenic causes (Ouslander, 1982). Respiration is the first and most effective defence against systemic, acid–base imbalances, of which there are four categories, acidosis and alkalosis, each of which may be due to metabolic or respiratory factors. Table 10.3 shows the values of pH, bicarbonates and pCO_2 in each of these conditions.

Table 10.3   Acidosis and alkalosis

	pH	$NaCO_3^-$ (mEq/l)	pCO_2
Metabolic acidosis	< 7.30	< 10	< 35
Respiratory acidosis	< 7.35	> 20	> 45
Metabolic alkalosis	> 7.45	> 30	< 55
Respiratory alkalosis	> 7.45	15–25	< 30

(Adapted from Plum and Posner, 1975)

Metabolic acidosis can occur relatively easily in the diabetic, who forgets his insulin-therapy, even though he maintains a proper diet. Psychic disturbances are already evident with a blood sugar of 250 mg% and the eventual ketonic bodies aggravate the pattern. High blood urea nitrogen (BUN) is another important cause of stupor or mental slowing, not infrequently due to reduced kidney filtration. However, there are individual variations, because some patients have disturbances of orientation even at 60 mg% of BUN, while others at 90 mg% do not. This leads us to think that a high BUN is connected with other factors, still unclear. In haemodialysis the clinical state improves, even though a high BUN can persist, and vice versa. Other causes of metabolic acidosis are rare, such as anoxic lactic acidosis and poisoning by acid substances, swallowed by mistake, as sometimes happens to elderly people living alone.

Respiratory acidosis, as opposed to the metabolic form, accompanies hyper-ventilation with a blood pH below 7.35, but with hypercapnia and normal bicarbonates. It may occur in the aged as a result of lung problems, but may also be due to reduced strength of the respiratory muscles. Besides the peripheral disturbances of respiration, we should remember the central ones, such as Pickwick's syndrome, when it is associated with obesity. This syndrome is a sleep apnoea-hypersomnia. The excessive somnolence seems to compensate for repeated awakening at night. It is a primary hypoventilation, but mechanical obstruction of the trachea can also play a role during sleep.

On the other hand, in respiratory alkalosis, the pH is above 7.45 and the hypocapnia coexists with a high percentage of bicarbonates. There are many causes and almost all are of a geriatric nature. They include long illnesses with hyperventilation, porta-cava encephalopathy, Gram-negative infections aggra-vated by fever and dehydration, salicylic intoxication which can occur in elderly patients with continuous articular pains and prolonged hyperventilation, in response to heat or to psychogenic factors.

Lastly, among disturbances of the acid-base balance we should mention the metabolic alkalosis. This is characterized by a pH above 7.45 and a large increase in bicarbonates. The condition may be due to the abuse of diuretics or to the excessive ingestion of alkalis, such as bicarbonate, by patients suffering from ulcer. Such practices are now less common, but the elderly are attached to old remedies, even when they have become obsolete. Other causes are Cushing's syndrome, due to prolonged steroid therapy, hormone-secreting lung carcinoma and also primary hyperaldosteronism. Metabolic alkalosis rarely presents in an acute manner, contrary to the other three forms of acid-base imbalance. As a result it can be an insidious cause of cognitive disturbances, sometimes attributed to cerebrovascular insufficiency. Hypothyroidism can also be a cause of stupor and coma especially in cold climates (Impallomeni, 1980).

In their daily work, geriatricians have to be ready to recognize hypoglycaemia in patients who for whatever reason have skipped a meal but continued the treatment, or who have absent-mindedly taken their hypoglycaemic pills twice. From this point of view, hypoglycaemic drugs are more dangerous for the aged than insulin itself and should be trusted only to extremely reliable patients or administered only in nurse-assisted conditions. Asthenia, perspiration and slight initial confusion must be promptly interpreted by the non-medical staff who care for these patients. They must be able to administer sugar as soon as possible, without confusing the symptoms with spontaneous and transitory vertigo, which

easily occurs in hypertensive older people. A marked confusional state, sometimes even reaching stupor, easily occurs through the use of sedative drugs
reinforced by a few glasses of wine or spirits. The risk associated with the use of
benzodiazepines in the elderly person who is sensitive to it are too high, and
unacceptable. This is demonstrated by the long sequences of iatrogenic beta in the
EEG, even after the withdrawal of the treatment, thus indicating the strength of
binding with the specific receptors. The use of tranquillizers can also facilitate
sleep apnoea and impair brain oxygenation (Kripke et al., 1982).

The precise rituals of nocturnal preparation, the worry of eventual insomnia
and the rigid behaviour of old habits make the aged faithful consumers of minor
tranquillizers and hypnotics. In demented patients, drugs such as tioridazine or
promethazine are preferred for protection against insomnia and nocturnal agitation, because they do not induce extrapyramidal signs at the usual dosage. The
tendency of elderly subjects to use hypnotics should be discouraged. Instead of
authoritarian prohibition, supportive discussion with the subject may have the
required tranquillizing effect, especially if it is reinforced with a placebo. It is
difficult to free an aged person from his disorders, but it is easy to create new ones
that are even worse.

We shall not deal in detail here with cerebral tumours and inflammatory
processes, because they are not problems of special concern in the elderly.
However, it is important to remember where tumours are concerned that the
surgical conditions are different. The removal of meningiomas is fatal in half of all
cases, although they are benign (Papo, 1983). The case for an operation must
therefore be carefully evaluated. Where cranial traumas are concerned, subdural
haematoma is sometime a serendipitous discovery in the CT scan. The incident
responsible for the haematoma may have been forgotten or minimized. The space
left by abiotrophic processes accounts for the long latency in the appearance of
clinical signs. Long-term use of anti-coagulant or platelet anti-aggregating drugs
can be risk factors for haematoma. The surgical prognosis is not correlated with
the length of clinical history, nor to the size of the haematoma, but to the patient's
age and the type of haematoma. The preoperative level, general state and the
intracranial complications (Sprung et al., 1984) are of importance in determining
suvival. A history of trauma is found in 66% of subdural haematomas and surgical
intervention has a successful outcome in 84% of cases. Intracerebral haematomas
are more frequent in elderly subjects than in the young: i.e. 47% vs. 26% (Karimi-
Nejad and Tritz, 1984). The case records of these authors show that age increases
the mortality in the case of moderately severe craniocerebral injury by 16–20%.
The highest mortality, 89%, strikes patients suffering from extra- and intracerebral mixed haematoma, while the outcome is less favourable in open head
traumas than closed head injuries.

REFERENCES

Agid, Y., Ruberg, M., Dubois, B., Pillon, B., and Javoy-Agid, F. (1985). Parkinsonism
    and dementia. *J. Neurol.*, 232 (Suppl.), 26.
Agnoli, A., Baldassarre, M., Ceci, E., Del Roscio, S., and Cerasoli, A. (1980). Aging and

extrapyramidal syndromes (parkinsonism). In G. Barbagallo-Sangiorgi and A. N. Exton-Smith (Eds), *The Aging Brain*. New York: Plenum Press, pp. 323–342.

Alexander, M. P., and Geschwind, N. (1984). Dementia in the elderly. In M. L. Albert (Ed.), *Clinical Neurology of Aging*. Oxford: Oxford University Press, pp. 254–276.

Baas, H., and Fischer, P. A. (1985). Sebaceous gland dysfunction in Parkinsonism. Excretion rate and composition of skin-surface lipids. *J. Neurol.*, 232 (Suppl.), 66.

Battistini, N., and Passero, S. (1985). Correlations between cerebral blood flow and brain atrophy in demented and non-demented patients. *J. Neurol.*, 232 (Suppl.), 158.

Berg, L. (1985). Does Alzheimer's disease represent an exaggeration of normal aging? *Arch. Neurol.*, 42, 737–739.

Boller, F., Goldstein, G., Dorr, C., Kim, Y., Moossy, J., Richey, E., Wagener, D., and Wolfson, S. K. (1984). Alzheimer and related dementias: a review of current knowledge. In G. Goldstein (Ed.), *Advances in Clinical Neuropsychology*. New York: Plenum Press, pp. 89–125.

Brody, J. A. (1985). Prospects for an ageing population. *Nature*, 315, 463–466.

Busse, E., and Simpson, D. (1983). Depression and antidepressant in the elderly. *Journal Clin. Psychiat.*, 44, 35–39.

Busse, E. W. (1985). The next twenty years: medical science and the practice of geriatrics. In C. M. Gaitz and T. Samorajski (Eds). *Aging 2000: Our Health Care Destiny*. New York: Springer-Verlag, pp. 17–26.

Dupont, E. (1980). Parkinson's disease and essential tremor: differential diagnostic and epidemiological aspects. In U.K. Rinne, M. Klinger, G. Stamm (Eds), *Parkinson's Disease*. New York: Elsevier-North Holland, pp. 165–179.

Fieschi, C., Orzi, F., Pocchiari, M., Nardini, M., Rocchi, F., Asher, D., Gibbs, C., and Gajdusek, D. (1983). Creutzfeld-Jakob disease in the province of Siena: two cases transmitted to monkeys. *Ital. J. Neurol. Sci.*, 4, 61–64.

Folstein, M. F., Folstein, S. E., and McHugh, P. R. (1975). Mini mental state. A practical method for grading the cognitive state of patients for the clinician. *J. Psychiat. Research*, 12, 189–198.

Francolini, P., Giaquinto, S., Massi, G., and Nolfe, G. (1985). Quantitative study of action tremor in various patient categories. *Ital. J. Neurol. Sci.*, 6, 67–73.

Giovannini, P., Scigliano, G., Grassi, M. P., Carella, F., Parati, E., and Caraceni, T. (1983). Bromocriptine-lisuride cross tolerance. *Ital. J. Neurol. Sci.*, 1, 129–130.

Gordon, E. B., and Sim, M. (1967). The EEG in presenile dementia. *J. Neurol. Neurosurg. Psychiat.*, 30, 285–291.

Gottfries, C. G. (1985). Rationale for the use of therapeutic agents in affective disorders (AD) and senile dementia of the Alzheimer type (SDAT). In C. M. Gaitz and T. Samorajski (Eds). *Aging 2000: Our Health Care Destiny*. New York: Springer-Verlag, pp. 327–338.

Gottfries, C. G., Adolfsson, R., Aquilonius, S. M., Carlsson, A., Oreland, L., Svenner-Holm, L., and Winblad, B. (1980). Parkinsonism and dementia disorders of Alzeheimer type: similarities and differences. In U.K. Rinne, M. Klinger, G. Stamm (Eds), *Parkinson's Disease*. New York: Elsevier–North Holland, pp. 197–208.

Growdon, J. H. (1985). Clinical profiles in Alzheimer's disease. In C. G. Gottfries (Ed.), *Normal Aging, Alzheimer's Disease and Senile Dementia*. Bruxelles: Editions de l'Université, pp. 213–218.

Guidetti, B., and Gagliardi, F. M. (1980). Dementia due to normal pressure hydrocephalus. In G. Barbagallo-Sangiorgi and A. N. Exton-Smith (Eds), *The Aging Brain*. New York: Plenum Press, pp. 161–177.

Gurian, B., and Auerbach, S. H. (1984). Psychiatric syndromes of old age. In M. L. Albert (Ed.), *Clinical Neurology of Aging*. Oxford: Oxford University Press, pp. 298–309.

Haan, J. (1983). Epilepsien und epileptische Anfalle im Alter. *Z. Gerontol.*, 16, 168–173.

Heston, L. L., Matri, A. R., Anderson, V. E., and White, J. (1981). Dementia of the

Alzheimer type: clinical genetics, natural history, and associated conditions. *Arch. Gen Psychiatry*, 38, 1085–1090.

Hietanen, M., and Teravainen, H. (1985). Motor disability vs. depression in Parkinson's disease. *J. Neurol.* 232 (Suppl.), 26.

Impallomeni, M. G. (1980). Central nervous system disturbances in myxoedema. In G. Barbagallo-Sangiorgi and A. N. Exton-Smith (Eds), *The Aging Brain*. New York: Plenum Press, pp. 179–193.

Johannesson, G., Hagberg, B., Gustafson, L., and Ingvar, D. H. (1979). EEG and cognitive impairment in presenile dementia. *Acta Neurol. Scand.*, 59, 225–240.

Jørg, J., and Schneider, A. (1985). Prognosis of normal pressure hydrocephalus. *J. Neurol.* 232 (Suppl.), 122.

Karimi-Nejad, A., and Tritz, W. (1984). Sequelae and prognosis of craniocerebral trauma in elderly people. *Adv. Neurosurg.*, 12, 212–215.

Katzman, R. (1983). Overview: demography, definitions and problems. In R. Katzman and R. D. Terry (Eds), *The Neurology of Aging*. Philadelphia, F. A. Davis Co., pp. 1–14.

Khachaturian, Z. S. (1985). Diagnosis of Alzheimer's disease. *Arch. Neurol.*, 42, 1097–1105.

Kolata, G. (1983). Clues to Alzheimer's disease emerge. *Science*, 219, 941–942.

Kolata, G. (1984). New neurons form in adulthood. *Science*, 224, 1325–1326.

Kripke, D. F., Ancoli Israel, S., and Okudaira, N. (1982). Sleep apnea and nocturnal myoclonus in the elderly. *Neurobiol. Aging*, 3, 329–336.

Lechi, A., Tedeschi, F., Mancia, D., Pietrini, V., Tagliavini, F., Terzano, M. G., and Trabattoni, G. (1983). Creutfeld–Jakob disease: clinical EEG and neuropathological findings in a cluster of eleven patients. *Ital. J. Neurol. Sci.*, 4, 47–59.

Lesser, J., Swihart, A., Beller, S., and Reed, K. (1985). Paraphrenia: preliminary results of neuropsychological testing. *Gerontologist*, 25 (Suppl.), 218.

Liston, E. H. (1979). Clinical findings of presenile dementia. *J. Nerv. Ment. Dis.*, 167, 337–342.

Loeb, C. (1980). Clinical diagnosis of multi-infarct dementia. In L. Amaducci, A. N. Davison and P. Antuono (Eds), *Aging*, vol. 13. New York: Raven Press, pp. 251–260.

Loeb, C., and Gandolfo, C. (1983). Diagnostic evaluation of degenerative and vascular dementia. *Stroke*, 14, 399–401.

Meyer, J. S., Kitagawa, Y., Tanahashi, N., Kandula, P., Rose, J. E., and Grossman, R. G. (1985). Dementia associated with normal pressure hydrocephalus. *J. Neurol.*, 232 (Suppl.), 122.

Mølsa, P. K., Paljarvi, L., Rinne, J. O., and Sakø, E. (1985). Accuracy of clinical diagnosis in patients with dementia. *J. Neurol.* 232 (Suppl.), 82.

Mormont, C. (1984). The influence of age and depression on intellectual and memory performance. *Acta Psychiat. Belg.*, 84, 127–134.

Muramoto, O. (1984). Selective reminding in normal and demented aged people: auditory verbal versus visual spatial task. *Cortex*, 20, 461–478.

Nakamura, S. (1982). Anthropological, behavioral and psychological factors in neuronal aging. In R. D. Terry, C. L. Bolis and G. Toffano (Eds), *Aging*, vol. 18. New York: Raven Press, pp. 197–207.

Nishihara, Y., and Ishii, N. (1985). Pathological study of demented old people. *J. Neurol.* 232 (Suppl.), 178.

Ouslander, J. G. (1982). Illness and psychopathology in the elderly. *Psych. Clin. North America*, 5, 145–148.

Papo, I. (1983). Intracranial meningiomas in the CT scan era. *Acta Neurochir.*, 67, 195–204.

Parnetti, L., Ciuffetti, G., Signorini, E., and Senin, U. (1985). Memory impairment in the elderly: a three-year follow-up. *Arch. Gerontol. Geriat.*, 4, 91–100.

Pinessi, L., Rainero, I., Asteggiano, G., Ferrero, P., Tarenzi, L., and Bergamasco, B.

(1984). Primary dementias: epidemiologic and sociomedical aspects. *Ital. J. Neurol. Sci.*, 5, 51–55.

Plum, F., and Posner, J. B. (1975). *Diagnosis of Stupor and Coma*. Philadelphia: Davies Co.

Rinne, J. O., Rinne, J. K., Laakso, K., and Lønnberg, P. (1985). Dopamine D-1 receptors in the parkinsonian brain. *J. Neurol.*, 232 (Suppl.), 10.

Rocca, W. A., Amaducci, L., and Schoenberg, B. S. (1986). Epidemiology of clinically diagnosed Alzheimer's disease. *Ann. Neurol.*,19, 415–424.

Roman, G. C. (1985) Lacunar dementia: a small artery form of vascular dementia. *J. Neurol.*, 232 (suppl.), 82.

Soininen, H., Jolkkonen, J., Ylinen, A., Halonen, T., Laulumaa, V., and Riekkinen, P. J. (1985). Cerebrospinal fluid cholinesterase and somatostatin in Parkinson's disease: relation to dementia. *J. Neurol.*, 232, (Suppl.), 26.

Sprung, C., Collmann, H., Kazner, E., and Duisberg, R. (1984). Chronic subdural hematoma in geriatric patients. Factors affecting prognosis. *Adv. Neurosurg.*, 12, 204–211.

Stern, G. M. (1980). Current adjuvant to levodopa therapy. In U.K. Rinne, M. Klinger and G. Stamm (Eds), *Parkinson's Disease*. New York: Elsevier-North Holland, pp. 357–361.

Tohgi, H. (1985). Etiology and pathogenesis of dementia due to cerebrovascular disease. *J. Neurol.*, 232 (Suppl.), 62.

Tomlinson, B. E., Blessed, G., and Roth, M. I. (1970). Observations in the brains of demented old people. *J. Neurol. Sci.*, 11, 205–242.

Wells, C. E. (1982). Pseudodementia and the recognition of organicity. In D. F. Benson and D. Blumer (Eds), *Psychiatric Aspects of Neurological Disease*, vol. 2. New York: Grune & Stratten, pp. 167–178.

Wertheimer, J. (1984). Brain deterioration: clinical pictures and manifestations. In F. C. A. Visentin (Ed.), *Cerebral Decay*. Milano: Farmitalia, Carlo Erba, pp. 29–88.

Williamson, J. (1980). Depression and its management. In G. Barbagallo-Sangiorgi and A. N. Exton-Smith (Eds), *The Aging Brain*. New York: Plenum Press, 205–216.

Wiszniewski, H. M., Merz, G. S., Wen, G. Y., Iqbal, K. Grundke-Iqbal, I. (1985). Morphology and biochemistry of Alzheimer's disease. In J. T. Hutton and A. D. Kenny (Eds), *Senile Dementia of the Alzheimer Type*. New York: A. R. Liss, pp. 163–274.

Yesavage, J. A., Brink, T. L., Rose, T. L., Lum, O., Huang, V. Adey, M., and Von Leirer, O. (1983). Development and validation of a geriatric depression screening scale: a preliminary report. *J. Psychiat. Res.*, 17, 37–49.

Yoshimasu, F., Yasui, M. Yoshida, H., Yoshida, S., Uebayashi, Y., Yase, Y., Gajdusek, D. C., and Chen, K. M. (1985). Aluminium in Alzheimer's disease in Japan and Parkinsonism-Dementia in Guam. *J. Neurol.* 232 (Suppl.), 61.

CHAPTER 11

Cognitive drugs

Pharmacology holds out the hope of new forms of treatment for cognitive disorders. Many problems remain and progress depends on basic research and better understanding of the patient's condition.

It must be said at the outset that neurobiology has yet to come up with the elixir of life. The science has provided no indication of how to reverse or even slow down the normal aging of the brain. Nevertheless pharmacological treatments may be valuable when cognitive impairment is due to other factors. Unfortunately the pharmacopoeia contains many useless remedies which only lull the physician into a false sense of security, obscuring deeper and more reasonable intervention (Macdonald and Macdonald, 1982).

The elderly are avid consumers of drugs and enthusiastic followers of endless therapies. Compounds in aqueous solution are particularly popular, allowing the meticulous ceremony of drop counting. The increasing proportion of elderly people in the Western world obviously accounts for industrial interest in this field. This trend is not an undesirable one because commercial investment will support basic as well as applied research, contributing to public knowledge and the development of centres of learning. Although private concerns do not support research for philanthropic reasons, their injection of funding in this field is welcome because Governments are not spending enough to find solutions to the problems of Alzheimer's disease and the other causes of mental deterioration in old age (Hollister, 1985).

There is no treatment for Alzheimer's disease and as yet no indication of when science will provide us with a means of controlling the third member of the triad: depression, delirium and dementia. However, even the most pessimistic observer would have to admit that we know a great deal more about the basic mechanism than we did even a few years ago. Hope for the future must lie in the further development of that knowledge. In this chapter we shall look at the main areas of pharmacological research that are relevant to the cognitive impairments of old age.

Drugs which affect brain circulation are widely used. They are classified as follows (Passeri and Cucinotta, 1980).

1) drugs with a mainly eumetabolic action
2) drugs with a vasoactive and eumetabolic action
3) drugs with a mainly alpha-blocker action
4) drugs with a mainly beta-facilitating action
5) drugs with a mainly myolytic action

Many of these are not placebo preparations. They can usefully be applied in the care of mild subjective symptoms such as headache, dizziness, drowsiness which have a circulatory basis or to the more serious consequences of cerebrovascular diseases. However, they are not really 'cognitive drugs'. This title should be reserved for those drugs which bring about positive changes in higher mental function, that is to say changes which are considered useful in medical treatment. Recent reviews present reasons for both pessimism and optimism (Cherkin and Riege, 1983; Goodnick and Gershon, 1983; Galizia, 1984).

At the present time, three lines of research are in progress with relevance to the aging brain. The first is focused on neurotransmitters. Since a fall of choline-acetyltransferase is known to occur in Alzheimer's disease, an obvious approach is to stimulate acetylcholine synthesis. Precursors such as choline, deanol and lecithin, have been given to patients but proof of positive results is still lacking. Physostigmine and also arecholine, a post-synaptic cholinergic agonist, have been used in an attempt to counteract the breakdown of the neurotransmitter. Although muscarinic receptors are known to survive the brain wasting of Alzheimer's disease, the final outcome of these trials has been disappointing, in spite of isolated positive results (Gottfries, 1985). Where the dementia or cognitive disorders can be shown to involve dopaminergic loss it might be expected that L-DOPA might be of value as it is in Parkinson's disease. However trials have been disappointing. The addition of an agonist, such as bromocriptine and lisuride, has not improved the therapeutic outcome. However some positive effects have been obtained, especially at the emotional level, in patients treated with alaproclate, a drug which acts selectively on the re-uptake of serotonin in the synaptic cleft (Gottfries, 1985).

Acetyl-L-carnitine is a natural compound having a role in the homeostasis of cellular acetylation (carnitine is called a 'geriatric vitamin' by Tener, 1985). It has been shown to bring about improvements in cognitive and memory functions of senile patients in a double-blind study (Agnoli, 1985). Alzheimer patients also show a trend toward normalization of the EEG spectrum after three months' therapy on a dosage of 1.5 g/day, with a reduction of the (delta+theta)/alpha ratio, compared to placebo (Giaquinto, unpublished observations). Positive effects induced by acetyl-L-carnitine were seen in rats with parallel histological and histochemical changes. Lipofuscin deposition in hippocampal pyramidal neurons and demyelinization in cortical 'lamina quinta' and sciatic nerve were reduced (Angelucci and Ramacci, 1985). This drug also prevents both the behavioural and electrophysiological changes of drug-induced parkinsonian-like syndrome in the monkey (Onofrj et al., 1986).

A second research trend focuses on the so-called 'nootropic' drugs, which have a selective effect on neurons. Their use in dementia is suggested by their telencephalic site of action, their protective effect on ATP and by remarkable results in animals. The first nootropic drug to appear on the market was piracetam, a gabaergic compound. A new nootropic drug, oxiracetam, appears to be effective in restoring the EEG profile in fronto-temporal regions in patients previously treated with diazepam (Giaquinto et al., 1984). Studies are in progress on demented patients with the assistance of Positron Emitted Tomography.

The third line of research concerns neuromodulation in the domain of the phospholipids. It has been suggested that drugs which have direct action on synapses are likely to be unprofitable in demented patients because of the severity of their side-effects. It is held that the modulation of receptors may provide a more practical approach. The gangliosides are compounds that may work in this manner.

Psychostimulants, which were widely used in the past (pentylenetetrazole, methylphenidate) are now obsolete because they lack beneficial effects and have unwanted vegetative side-effects. The well-known Gerovital, i.e. procaine in a suitable preparation for intramuscular administration, is also obsolete. Since local inactivation occurs, negligible amounts of the drug reach the central nervous system. Hyperbaric oxygen was once thought to improve cerebral oxygenation, but the results have been disappointing. Moreover, it may worsen the condition of the patient who has already had an ischaemic cerebrovascular attack.

The field of experimental therapy for cognitive defects has been criticized for its failure to adopt a common protocol of investigation. It has been argued that the patchy results obtained so far are due to three problems: a) the groups of patients are not homogeneous, and often unselected; b) instrumentation for measurement is inadequate in many cases; c) the approach is naive, because it is not possible to single out one neurotransmitter system as the primary locus of impairment in dementia (Agnoli, 1985).

According to the critics, the ideal methodology would tailor the treatment for each patient after careful investigations, including biochemical studies of the spinal fluid. Supporting the idea of combined treatment, it has also been suggested (Meier-Ruge, 1983) that glycolytic and tricarboxylic acid turnover should be improved, since this seems to be the most important metabolic system in acetylcholine synthesis.

The criticism that research in this field lacks strict and standard protocols is valid. However simple or complex the pharmacological model under evaluation, an attempt should be made to match the groups properly on the basis of medical and social history, to investigate the medical condition of subjects thoroughly and to design the experiments with proper controls, double-blind, and with statistical analysis. There are bound to be variations in terms of what is locally possible, but the following list of factors to take into account is put forward as a basis for discussion:

Subject variables: patient, outpatient, normal; age, sex, socioeconomic group, income, home town, living-together, education, job.

Illness: normal aging, AD/SD, MID, other diseases, beginning, evolution, cognitive damage, risk factors.

Environment: stimulation, indifference, hostility, recent changes of house, recent losses, climate, diet, intoxications.

Internal medicine: subjective symptoms, heart and vessels, lungs, liver, kidney, general metabolism.

Neurology: clinical signs, CT scan, CBF, PET, NMR, EEG, event-related potentials, spinal fluid, biopsy, neuropsychological testing, behavioural videotape.

Psychiatry: testing for anxiety and depression, Rorschach.

Parallel therapies: neuroleptics, antidepressants, nootropics, vasoactive and antiparkinson drugs.

Experimental design: frequency of observations, place, time, statistics, observers and judges.

Drugs: dosage, administration, duration, double-blind, monitoring, enhancement by training.

Further questions may be posed. What is the best neuropsychological method of testing? What are the most reliable electrophysiological correlates? What are the proper markers in the cerebral spinal fluid? What is the minimal requirement for a therapy to be considered effective?

Neurochemistry and neuropharmacology still have a long way to go before they make any major impact on therapy for cognitive disorders. Spectacular results have not yet been achieved, though there is hope that improvements will come not only from developments in these sciences but also in improvements in diagnosing the conditions to which drug treatments can be applied. No possibility should be neglected for alleviating the burden of Alzheimer's disease and other forms of mental decay, moving this time from care to cure.

Chemistry was born in the 16th century, but four more centuries elapsed before the first antiepileptic molecule was discovered. Nowadays, more than two thirds of all epileptic patients are successfully controlled by medical therapy, whereas the great neurologists of the 19th century were unable to offer any effective treatment for the condition. For them, epilepsy was as intractable as dementia appears to us today.

Any effective medical treatment for Alzheimer's disease must concentrate on halting or reversing its highly progressive course. This raises an important and fundamental problem. If an effective drug were discovered which immediately restored the impaired neurochemical milieu, the reinstalled memory stores of the patient would be devoid of previous information, and the mind would be ill prepared for language, thinking, and abstract reasoning. This would be of little benefit to the patient. It follows that each pharmacological treatment needs to be carried out in parallel with neuropsychological training.

REFERENCES

Agnoli, A. (1985). Discussion on the therapeutical effect of acetyl-L-carnitine in psycho-organic syndrome and senile dementia. *IVth World Congress of Biological Psychiatry*, Philadelphia, 1985.

Angelucci, L., and Ramacci, M. T. (1985). Acetyl-L-carnitine: neuropharmacological potentialities in senescent rats. *IVth World Congress of Biological Psychiatry*, Philadelphia, 1985.

Cherkin, A., and Riege, W. H. (1983). Multimodal approach to pharmacotherapy of senile amnesias. In J. Cervos-Navarro and H. I. Sarkander (Eds), *Aging*, vol. 21. New York: Raven Press, pp. 415–435.

Galizia, V. (1984). Pharmacotherapy of memory loss in the geriatric patient. *Drug Intell. Clin. Pharmacol.*, 18, 784–791.

Giaquinto, S., Nolfe, G., and Vitali, S. (1984). EEG changes induced by oxiracetam on diazepam-medicated volunteers. *Clin. Neuropharmacol.*, 7, 786–787.

Goodnick, P. J., and Gershon, S. (1983). Chemotherapy of cognitive disorders. In D. Samuel, S. Algeri, S. Gershon, V. E. Grimm and G. Toffano (Eds), *Aging*, vol. 22. New York: Raven Press, pp. 349–361.

Gottfries, C. G. (1985). Rationale for the use of therapeutic agents in affective disorders (AD) and senile dementia of the Alzheimer type (SDAT). In C. M. Gaitz and T. Samorajski (Eds). *Aging 2000: Our Health Care Destiny*. New York: Springer-Verlag, pp. 327–338.

Hollister, L. E. (1985). Pharmacotherapy of mental disorders of old age. In C. M. Gaitz and T. Samorajski (Eds). *Aging 2000: Our Health Care Destiny*. New York: Springer-Verlag, pp. 303–315.

Macdonald, E. T., and Macdonald, J. B. (1982). *Drug Treatment in the Elderly*. New York: John Wiley & Sons.

Meier-Ruge, W. (1983). New prospects in neuropharmacology of senile dementia. In J. Cervos-Navarro and H. I. Sarkander (Eds), *Aging*, vol. 21. New York: Raven Press, pp. 391–399.

Onofrj, M. C., Felice, M., Ghilardi, M., Bodis-Wollner, I. G., and Glover, A. A. (1986). L-Acetylcarnitine (LAC) prevents MPTP-induced parkinsonian-like syndrome (PS) in the monkey. *Neurology*, 36 (Suppl. 1), 96.

Passeri, M., and Cucinotta, D. (1980). Principles and methods of evaluating mental disorders in the aged and the modifications following drug administration. In G. Barbagallo-Sangiorgi and A. N. Exton-Smith (Eds), *The Aging Brain*. New York: Plenum Press, 275–293.

Tener, G. M. (1985). Ageing society. *Nature*, 316, 386.

CHAPTER 12

Neuropsychological training

Programmes of stimulation can take advantage of neural plasticity to improve cognitive performance even in the elderly.

Mental exercise on tasks of increasing speed has positive effects on cognitive ability in the elderly, especially when it is combined with treatment on 'nootropic' drugs. Psychopharmacological studies like these are in progress all over the world in the search for methods to restore the communication channels of the central nervous system to bring about cognitive, affective and behavioural recovery. The most important period of development occurs in childhood when the initial patterns of connectivity are established. Even in this period the changes are not passively neurochemical. The child's brain contains structures whose role in language is genetically predetermined, but the child will grow up without speech unless he is trained through communication with others. Similarly, the structures for reading and writing are present but he will remain illiterate unless taught to use them. In exactly the same way, a powerful computer remains impotent until programmed. We must not expect drugs to restore function passively in the elderly either; they will have to be administered within the framework of a treatment plan that includes training and cognitive and behavioural techniques if they are to do any good.

Training has proved very effective in the elderly, even though it is normally presumed that the capacity for development is reduced and the ability of the system to cope with information is slowed. Neuropsychological training can give more self-reliance to the elderly, just as reality therapy can affect small improvements in the daily life of the demented patients to lighten his burden.

The potential for obtaining positive effects from training rests on a number of important biological phenomena. To begin with, it is well known that peripheral axons retain the capacity of regeneration in the adult, and a continuous process of regression and renewal takes place at peripheral synapses (Giacobini, 1982). There is a positive balance between degeneration and regeneration in a process of constant rejuvenation and plasticity. This process begins to slow down in elderly people, but does not disappear. Its character is modified too. As we saw in Chapter 9, the terminals at the motor endplate increase in number with more arborization, more synaptic vesicles and more receptors for acetylcholine.

Studies of metabolism markers in the rat (Benzi et al., 1980) demonstrated that the level of some enzymes fluctuates with a periodicity like that of a dampened oscillation. This indicates the existence of natural renewal processes which might be capable of enhancement using appropriate techniques. Evidence that it is possible to increase the metabolism of catecholamines comes from a study of the effect of external stimulation in moderately deteriorated patients. Groups of 4–5 subjects underwent two weekly sessions of motor and cognitive exercise each lasting an hour and also manipulations of emotional behaviour. The cerebrospinal fluid showed an increase in the level of homovanillic acid, which represents one of the terminal metabolites of catecholamine breakdown. The result was attributed to both dendritic and synaptic growth (Karlsson et al., 1984).

In recent years several studies have demonstrated that selective lesions, which partially damage the neuronal input to the dendritic tree, induce the sprouting of residual terminals. The sprouts establish new synaptic connections in place of those which have been lost (Cotman et al., 1981). The process is called reactive synaptogenesis and allows the remodelling of new neuronal systems.

Another mechanism of plasticity in the central nervous system is the growth of dendrites which does not seem to be affected by aging. In fact, computerized microscopy has revealed that the dendritic trees in the second layer of the human hippocampus are larger in the normal elderly than in younger controls, and smallest in patients affected by primary dementia (Buell and Coleman, 1981). The greatest differences are observed at the level of the terminal segments of the dendritic tree at a moderate distance for the cell body, rather than at the proximal or distal extremes. The terminal parts of the dendrites have extensions or branchings, while the basal parts have only extensions. This finding is very interesting, because it shows that even in old age the phenomena of plasticity appear as well as those of regression. Even the rate of growth remains constant at the growth cone, 0.21 μm/year from 44 to 92 years.

It is not clear why development is concentrated at the apex: whether the neurochemical composition is different here or whether the input and thus stimulation occurs particularly at the level of the dendritic apex.

The importance of input on dendritic growth is demonstrated by other observations. If old rats are kept in an environment rich in stimuli, the dendrites of the third and fourth cortical layers grow longer than those in rats kept in isolation (Green et al., 1983). A period of 45 days is sufficient to cause significant differences in the dendrites of the third layer at 40 or at 140 μm from the cell body, and 40 μm from the cell body in the fourth layer.

Other evidence obtained from rats kept in isolation suggests that more N (*nubbin*) type dendrites, which are qualitatively different from normal, may be produced by the reduced stimulation (Diamond and Connor, 1984). In humans, environmental stimulation increases cerebral blood flow to levels significantly greater than that found in the elderly residents in institutions providing low levels of social stimulation (Kobayashi et al., 1984).

These lines of evidence suggest that stimulation has favourable effects on even elderly brains, especially on the proliferation of dendritic trees. Nevertheless the plastic and adaptive capacity for re-innervation in the central nervous system reduces as the years go by. The causes are not understood, but one of the factors so far identified is that the high level of glucocorticoid hormones slows down repair (Scheff et al., 1984). This observation is important in the therapy of acute vasculopathies, because the common use of steroids against cerebral oedema may disturb plasticity and so delay rehabilitation, if the treatment is protracted. Scheff et al. have also observed the behaviour of reactive synaptogenesis in the molecular layer of the hippocampus in the rat. Removing the entorhinal cortex that projects to the outer 3/4 of that layer, irregularity and reduction of synapses is noted after two days. In the fourth day, neosynaptogenesis begins, while astrocytes clean up the denervated areas. The reconstruction process reaches its peak after one month and is maintained at this level for a further six months. After this period, no further changes can be detected. An important factor in reactive synaptogenesis is the presence of a contingent of contralateral fibres.

Even the septal areas participate in the reconstruction with intense proliferation of septo-hippocampal cholinergic fibres. By measuring the enzymatic activity of synthesis (CAT) and of breakdown (AChE) it is deduced that there is actually an increased turnover. The pattern of degenerative products in aged animals is identical to that found in younger controls. The conclusion is that the pattern of entorhinal input to the hippocampus does not change with age. The patterns of AChE staining are also identical for the two age groups and only the amount of staining in the outer three fourths of the molecular layer is quantitatively different.

Anatomical regeneration is not the only process which affects recovery. An additional compensatory mechanism is suggested by the following experiments. A lesion of the lateral hypothalamus induces contralateral hemi-inattention in the rat. The same effect is obtained by a selective catecholaminergic neurotoxin (6-OHDA). The lesion is followed by recovery over the first five days. The recovery depends on the restoration of dopaminergic activity because it is facilitated by an agonist, the apomorphine, or by the implantation of dopaminergic neurons in the neostriatum. Since no anatomical changes are visible in the neostriatum, which receives afferent nerves from the injured hypothalamus, the recovery is attributed to restored dopaminergic activity, but only as far as the fifth day. Thereafter, the course of recovery is the same for both the physical lesions and the injection of 6-OHDA, so it is presumed that another mechanism intervenes, namely increased post-synaptic sensitivity (Marshall, 1984).

Further observations on rats indicate that lesions of the 90–95% dopaminergic areas of the mesencephalon causes cessation of spontaneous feeding. If force fed for some weeks, they recover their hunger drive maintaining weight without assistance. This phenomenon may be explained by a mechanism of adaptation, which is immediately effected, by which the remaining neurons within the affected area continue to receive sufficient input to maintain its function. This may be achieved by an increase in dopaminergic turnover with reduced re-uptake (Stricker and Zigmond, 1984).

The number of dopaminergic receptors declines with aging, yet it has been demonstrated that this receptor system is able to react to an agonist with negative feed-back on dopaminergic turnover and with an increase of sensitivity after a prolonged block (Algeri et al., 1982).

The dendrites, the antennae which provide nerve cells capable of up to 10,000 connections with other neurones, occupy a critical position in the mechanisms for processing information in the brain. In Chapter 4 we viewed the connectivity established by the dendritic trees as the hardware for an intracortical associative memory system. In addition to communication through synapses, there is the possibility that the dendrites exchange the information even more quickly by electrotonic conduction (Schmitt et al., 1981). Any involution of the dendrite would affect both systems, leading to the slowing of cognitive speed in the elderly. Conversely, training may exert its positive effects through maintenance and even development of dendritic fields. Specifically, training might lead to the establishment of synapses or to growth of the dendritic trees, enhancing speed and the capacity for data storage. Fig. 12.1 illustrates the various models of restoration so far put forward to account for repair and recovery in the nervous system: regeneration, dendritic growth, sprouting and branching, increase in presynaptic activity in turnover of transmitters, postsynaptic hypersensitivity, and the activation of silent lines.

The first part of this chapter has dealt with mechanisms that may be responsible for repair and recovery in the central nervous system because we cannot expect training to combat the decline associated with aging and disease unless some form of neural plasticity remains in the adult brain. Having seen that a number of different mechanisms remain operative which may serve this purpose, we can examine the claims that the elderly derive benefit from neuropsychological intervention. Many different strategies have been tried, and have been covered by reviews elsewhere (for example, Birren et al., 1983). We shall select only studies which exemplify the main factors affecting improvement in cognitive function in the elderly.

A test of inductive reasoning was the training task for a group of 60 women, average age 76 years, who were paid to participate in the study. The subjects had to find the relation between a series of letters and identity the odd one out. One group received help from specific instructions and another did not (Labouvie-

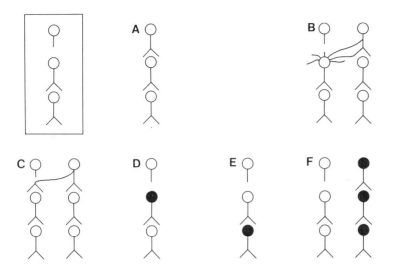

Fig. 12.1   Schematic drawing of reparative and adaptive mechanisms in the nervous system. Regeneration (A), sprouting, (B), branching (C), increased turnover (D), postsynaptic supersensitivity (E), activation of a silent line (F)

Vief and Gonda, 1976). The greatest effect of training has been seen in the group that received no help and therefore had to work out the strategy for themselves. The effect of training generalized to other tasks and indeed the procedure would have little practical value if the benefit were limited to the training task. Evidence for the transfer to other activities was provided by improvement in performance on Raven's Standard Progressive Matrices. The generalization to other tasks of the benefits derived from training has been shown to long outlast the period of training in the elderly (Sanders and Clawson Sanders, 1978). In this study improvement in performance was evident after initial training in a group of 34 volunteers, average age 72 years.

In a study of rehearsal strategies in tasks of free recall, it was found that a control group of elderly subjects, who were invited only to remember and to recall words from lists of categories, used simple strategies of iteration as an aid to recall. By contrast, a group trained to practice rehearsal and to recall the words by categories showed a very clear advantage, independent of the amount of simple rehearsal (Schmitt et al., 1981). The authors conclude that the recall is best in subjects trained to use elaborate strategies. Thus, the failure of elderly subjects to adopt an effective strategy is a production deficiency that can be overcome with appropriate training.

Training does not improve all tasks in the same way; for example, practice with the use of visual mediators does not help on face–name recall and practice with the use of association of images does not help on paragraph retention. However, there is no indication that any improvement in cognitive ability is reflected in improvement in the affective state of the elderly patient (Zarit et al., 1981).

A different approach has been adopted in studies designed to train subjects to process information presented tachistoscopically. In a group of subjects with an average age of 66 years, training with tachistoscopic stimuli brought about improvements not only in signal detection but in memory scanning and in visual discrimination over 50 hours of practice sessions (Salthouse and Somberg, 1982). With the dichoptic presentation of target and mask stimuli the interval necessary to escape masking was reduced by about 33 msec in 5 days of practice, even though the difference between the elderly group and young controls persisted (Hertzog et al., 1976). The capacity to increase the speed of central processing is confirmed by other studies in which operant conditioning is reinforced by monetary reward (Baron et al., 1983; Baron and Menich, 1985). These investigations provide interesting results because they reveal that motivation is as important as practice in bringing about improvement. The persistence of age differences even after training partially invalidates the 'disuse' theory of aging, because such differences should have been abolished. It accords with the theory only to the extent that it reveals the possibility of reversing the decline associated with aging.

The practice effect, common to the young and the elderly, applies to many other situations of repeated learning over time, as for example the verbal learning curves for Rey's test. Here the improvement due to practice can be greater than the differences due to age (Baron and Menich, 1985).

Studies made in our laboratory have shown that it is possible to modify reaction time and tachistoscopic threshold, elements which are regarded as measures of so-called fluid intelligence. For example, Fig. 12.2 shows the case of a 70-year-old subject trained twice each week for a total of eight sessions on a choice reaction time task. He had to distinguish between a target (a red frame subtending 8° for 18 msec) and a non-target stimulus (a blue frame). Two different decrements in choice reaction time are seen in the graph, of which the first is situation-specific and the second related to the real effect of training.

This is an example of an approach known as 'testing the limits' meaning to test the subjects to the limit of their cognitive abilities. This method is particularly effective in revealing age differences, reserve capacity, and changes due to compensation and plasticity. The fact that elderly patients may outscore young people when stretched to the limit in this way demonstrates the residual plasticity of the old brain (Baltes and Kliegl, 1986).

In general, recall improves if the method of loci is used in which the item to be remembered is associated with visual images from familiar locations (such as different places in the subject's house) reinforced with pleasant associations (Yesavage and Rose, 1984). However, the level of improvement obtained with this method diminishes in the elderly, possibly from a deficit of semantic elaboration or because of a deficit in retrieval or a difficulty in generating and recovering visual images.

The improved capacity for remembering lists of names or concepts is clearly a help with everyday tasks such as purchases, appointments and conversations.

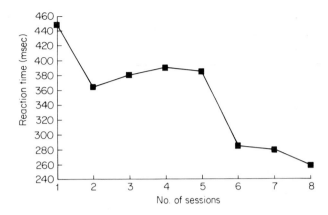

Fig. 12.2 Profile of performance in a 70-year-old subject, trained on a choice reaction task. The mean value at this age is 482 msec (SD 169). The first improvement is probably due to a familiarization with the experimental setting. The sharp improvement at the fifth session is the manifestation of better allocation of mental resources. The subject is trained during two sessions/week of 45 min duration each

Strategies involving the use of categorization, clustering and visual images have been investigated in subjects of various ages, who from the beginning make extensive use of high categorization and little use of imagery. Clustering and imagery capacity improves with training, but the strategy which provides the highest level of recall remains categorization (Rankin, 1984). However, the memory of elderly subjects for a specific task can be improved by training them on visual imagery. This facilitates one of the most difficult tasks for the aged, face–name recall, because it facilitates mental organization itself (Yesavage, 1985).

Other strategies recommended for the elderly subject include dwelling a little more on the material to be learned, allowing it to 'sink-in' and making a response to the material when it is first presented: this is the 'discovery' method, used in industrial training (Welford, 1985). With a minimum of preliminary instructions, a training follows in which the subject resolves the problem at his own speed and errors are minimized or corrected rapidly. In other words, subjects receive few verbal instructions and successively discover for themselves at their own pace the way to cope.

Personal computers will probably play an important future role in neuropsychological training of the elderly, providing continuous dialogue and interactive answers. The training must be long to provide adequate reinforcement and be sufficiently complex to maintain interest and involvement. It seems that procedures which do not permit the correction of mistakes favour quicker learning. An asymptote does not necessarily indicate that one has obtained optimal behaviour (Perone and Baron, 1983).

Training also has a favourable effect upon motor skill in both the normal elderly and those who are ill. For example, tremor induced by Parkinson's disease can be reduced when the patient has to master a task of visuomotor co-ordination. The improvement occurs gradually (Fig. 12.3) and is not solely due to practice.

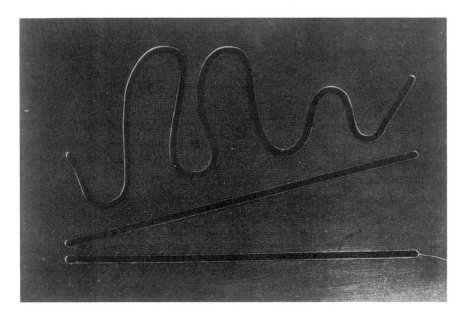

Fig. 12.3 Board for the study of action tremor. The subject has to slide a special metal stylus in the grooves. The panel has zero voltage and the stylus an anode voltage of 10 V. The test starts when the stylus passes in front of a photodiode hidden under the panel. Another photodiode automatically stops the clock at the end of the trial. Digital displays indicate total time, number of errors (contacts) and total time of contact. The subject resets the equipment after each trial and writes down the values indicated by the displays (from Francolini et al., 1985)

Patients become more aware of their abilities and less concerned about their motor performances in daily life. Effective motor training needs visual reinforcement and should be carried out without the presence of an observer. Relaxation, self-esteem and competence are then improved as in the task shown in Fig. 12.4. Reduction of tension is known to improve performance, because anxiety has a negative effect on attention and memory in the elderly (Yesavage and Jacob, 1984). Relaxation training is therefore also useful.

The assimilation of motor aspects during encoding (multimodal encoding) provides another strategy, like a contextual support which can be used by elderly subjects to improve their free recall (Backman and Nilsson, 1985). This method can reduce age differences.

As Willis and Schaie have observed (1985) 'training gain occurs at the level of the ability constructs and is not limited to a test-specific effect. In addition,

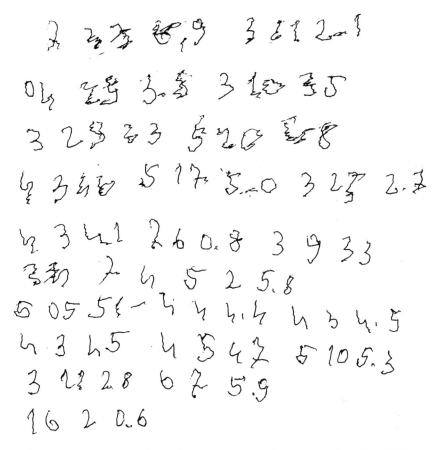

Fig. 12.4 Improvement of parkinsonian tremor with exercise (see Fig. 12.3). A women of age 72 under steady anticholinergic treatment. The session took 40 minutes

training was found particularly effective for subjects having experienced previous decline on the ability trained'. Neuropsychological training is different from the so-called reality orientation therapy because it deals with more complex cognitive events, demands high levels of performance, incorporates reinforcement, even of a monetary nature, or the expectation of an improvement in the health of the subject.

Reality orientation is a treatment for confused or demented patients (for a general background and for controlled studies, see Woods and Holden, 1982). Its detailed description is beyond the aims of this book as it is not generally beneficial for the normal elderly. On the other hand, it is worth noting that rehabilitation therapy can be used to help elderly subjects who have no evident cognitive damage but reduced motivation (Lewis, 1984). Lewis recommends engaging the patient emotionally, physically and mentally. It is necessary to individualize the treatment programme making the patient participate in the choice of activities and ensuring that health workers and families provide support. This intensive programme involves encouraging the subject in creative activities and in the use of recreational facilities in order to acquire interest, competence and usefulness.

Neuropsychological training and the techniques of rehabilitation benefit the patient only if they are offered within a socially meaningful context. The improvements in cognitive function observed in laboratory experiments may satisfy our scientific curiosity but they will not do the patient any good unless they have a bearing in his everyday life. In particular, it is easy for patients who have been intensively and exclusively studied for research to experience frustration and dejection when the project is over and they are no longer of interest. The clinical management of these patients must ensure that they take away an understanding of an important biological principle, that use brings functional efficiency and non-use brings defective function (Eccles, 1953).

REFERENCES

Algeri, S., Achilli, G., Cimino, M., Perego, C., Ponzio, F., and Vantani, G. (1982). Study on some compensatory responses of dopaminergic system in aging rats. *Exp. Brain Res.*, suppl. 5, 146–149.

Backman, L., and Nilsson, L. G. (1985). The avoidance of age differences in single-trial free recall. *Ann N.Y. Acad. Sci.*, 444, 523–524.

Baltes, P. B., and Kliegl, R. (1986). On the dynamics between growth and decline in the aging of intelligence and memory. In K. Poeck, H. J. Freund and H. Gaenshirt (Eds), *Neurology*. Berlin: Springer-Verlag, pp. 1–17.

Baron, A., and Menich, S. R. (1985). Age-related effects of temporal contingencies on response speed and memory: an operant analysis. *J. Gerontol.*, 40, 60–70.

Baron, A., Menich, S. R., and Perone, M. (1983). Reaction times of younger and older men and temporal contingencies of reinforcement. *J. Exp. Anal. Behav.*, 40, 275–287.

Benzi, G., Arrigoni, E., Dagani, F., Marzatico, F., Curti, D., Polgatti, M., and Villa, R. F. (1980). Drug interference on the age-dependent modification of the cerebral enzymatic activities related to energy transduction. In L. Amaducci, A. N. Davison and P. Antuono (Eds), *Aging*, vol. 3. New York: Raven Press, 113–117.

Birren, J. E., Cunningham, W. R., and Yamamoto, K. (1983). Psychology of adult development and aging. *Ann. Rev. Psychol.*, 34, 543–575.

Buell, S. J., and Coleman, P. D. (1981). Quantitative evidence for selective dendritic growth in normal human aging but not in senile dementia. *Brain Res.*, 214, 23–41.

Cotman, C. W., Nieto-Sampedro, M., and Harris, E. W. (1981). Synapse replacement in the adult nervous system of vertebrates. *Physiol. Rev.*, 61, 684–784.

Diamond, M. C., and Connor, J. R. (1984). Morphological measurements in the aging rat cerebral cortex. In S. W. Scheff (Ed.), *Aging and Recovery of Function in the Central Nervous System*. New York, Plenum Press, pp. 43–56.

Eccles, J. C. (1953). *The Neurophysiological Basis of Mind*. London: Oxford University Press.

Francolini, P., Giaquinto, S., Massi, G. and Nolfe, G. (1985). Quantitative study of action tremor in various patient categories. *Ital. J. Neurol. Sci.*, 6, 67–73.

Giacobini, E. (1982). Cellular and molecular mechanisms of aging in the nervous system: towards a unified theory of neuronal aging. In E. Giacobini, G. Filogamo, G. Giacobini and A. Vernadakis (Eds), *Aging*, vol. 20. New York: Raven Press, pp. 197–210.

Green, E. J., Greenough, W. T., and Schlumpf, B. E. (1983). Effects of complex or isolated environments on cortical dendrites of middle-aged rats. *Brain Res.* 264, 233–240.

Hertzog, C. K., Michael, V. W., and Walsh, D. A. (1976). The effect of practice on age differences in central perceptual processing. *J. Gerontol.*, 31, 428–433.

Karlsson, I., Brane, G., Melin, E., Nuth, A. L., and Rybo, E. (1984). Mental activation — Brain plasticity. *Clin. Neuropharmacol.*, 7 (suppl. 1), 336–337.

Kobayashi, S., Yamaguchi, S., Katsube, T., Kitani, M., Okada, K., and Kitamura, J. (1984). Influence of social environment factors on cerebral circulation and mental function in the normal aged. In C. Fieschi, G. L. Lenzi and C. Loeb (Eds), *Monograph in Neural Sciences*, vol. 11. Basel: Karger, pp. 163–168.

Labouvie-Vief, G., and Gonda, J. N. (1976). Cognitive strategy training and intellectual performance in the elderly. *J. Gerontol.*, 31, 327–332.

Lewis, C. B. (1984). Rehabilitation of the older person: a psychosocial focus. *Phys. Ther.*, 64, 517–522.

Marshall, J. F. (1984). Behavioral consequences of neuronal plasticity following injury to nigrostriatal dopaminergic neurons. In S. W. Scheff (Ed.), *Aging and Recovery of Function in the Central Nervous System*. New York, Plenum Press, pp. 101–128.

Perone, M., and Baron, A. (1983). Reduced age differences in omission errors after prolonged exposure to response pacing contingencies. *Dev. Psychol.*, 19, 915–923.

Rankin, J. L. (1984). Strategy use, recall, and recall organization in young, middle-aged, and elderly adults. *Exp. Aging Res.*, 10, 193–196.

Salthouse, T. A., and Somberg, B. L. (1982). Skilled performance: effects of adult age and experience in elementary processes. *J. Exp. Psychol.: General*, 111, 176–207.

Sanders, R. E., and Clawson-Sanders, J. A. (1978). Long-term durability and transfer of enhanced conceptual performance in the elderly. *J. Gerontol.*, 33, 408–412.

Scheff, S. W., Anderson, K., and Dekosky, S. T. (1984) Morphological aspects of brain damage in aging. In S. W. Scheff (Ed.), *Aging and Recovery of Function in the Central Nervous System*. New York, Plenum Press, pp. 57–85.

Schmitt, F. A., Murphy, M. D., and Sanders, R. E. (1981). Training older adult free recall rehearsal strategies. *J. Gerontol.*, 36, 329–337.

Stricker, E. W., and Zigmond, M. J. (1984). Recovery of function following brain damage: homeostasis at dopaminergic synapses. In G. Goldstein (Ed.), *Advances in Clinical Neuropsychology*. New York: Plenum Press, pp. 161–182.

Welford, A. T. (1985). Changes of performance with age: an overview. In N. Charness (Ed.), *Aging and Human Performance*. New York: John Wiley & Sons, pp. 333–369.

Willis, S. L., and Schaie, K. W. (1985). Cognitive training in a longitudinal sample. *Gerontologist*, 25 (suppl.), 10.

Woods, R. T., and Holden, U. P. (1982). Reality orientation. In B. Isaacs (Ed.), *Recent Advances in Geriatric Medicine*, 2. London: Churchill Livingstone, pp. 181–198.

Yesavage, J. A. (1985). Nonpharmacologic treatments for memory losses with normal aging. *Am. J. Psychiatry*, 142, 600–605.

Yesavage, J. A. and Rose, T. L. (1984). Semantic elaboration and the method of loci: a new trip for older learners. *Exp. Aging Res.*, 10, 155–159.

Yesavage, J. A., and Jacob, R. (1984). Effects of relaxation and mnemonics on memory, attention and anxiety in the elderly. *Exp. Aging Res.*, 10, 211–214.

Zarit, S. H., Cole, K. D., and Guider, R. L. (1981). Memory training strategies and subjective complaints of memory in the aged. *Gerontologist*, 21, 158–164.

CHAPTER 13

The social context of medical treatment

Medicine and Social Sciences eye one another with mutual distrust. Yet, Medicine without social interaction is hobbled and social intervention without Medicine is blind.

This chapter examines a number of social issues that affect the medical care of the elderly, and reveals the complex relationship that needs to exist between social and medical services. Frequently, however, the social science literature makes no reference to biomedical factors concerning the elderly. Yet it is important to be clear in dealing with 'the elderly' whether we are talking about those who have a disability, those who are over 65 or simply those in retirement. It is not possible to provide the right social measures without knowing to whom those measures must be adapted. In the great majority of cases, the important distinction is between self-sufficiency and non-self-sufficiency. But the first term may refer as much to the older person who is still lively, cultured and clever, as to the slightly deteriorated subject who is still able to look after himself. The second category may include people who, with medical intervention and adequate rehabilitation, could achieve 'small gains' (Williams, 1984) to modify the type of social intervention they require.

Intervention strategies for the aged (in the widest sense of the term) should be based on physical examination, cognitive evaluation and personality profiles, since these factors have an important influence on adjustment. Different character profiles have been identified even if the effects of different intervention strategies on the various sub-types are still unknown (Diana, 1983; Loebel and Eisdorfer, 1984; Silverstone, 1984). It is therefore clear that medicine and social services must proceed in parallel in an integrated and non-conflicting fashion.

We have seen that there is no general agreement on what is meant by aging, to the extent that it has not been definitively established whether mental decline is a necessary concomitant of aging. Geriatric scales, such as the SCAG (Table 13.1),

Table 13.1 SCAG scale

Assessment of clinical status

Rating key:
1 = not present   2 = very mild   3 = mild   4 = mild to moderate
5 = moderate   6 = moderately severe   7 = severe

1) Confusion
2) Mental alertness
3) Impairment of recent memory
4) Disorientation
5) Mood depression
6) Emotional lability
7) Self-care
8) Anxiety
9) Motivation–initiative
10) Irritability
11) Hostility
12) Bothersome
13) Indifference to surroundings
14) Unsociability
15) Uncooperativeness
16) Fatigue
17) Appetite
18) Dizziness
19) Overall impression of the patient

SCAG items	*Factors*
1, 2, 3, 4	Cognitive dysfunction
10, 11, 12, 15	Interpersonal relationships
5, 6, 8	Affective disorders
7, 9, 13, 14	Apathy
16, 17, 18	Somatic functioning

(from Sandoz Clinical Assessment Geriatric Rating Scale, simplified)

are useful instruments for social workers and for use in longitudinal studies although they have little or no value for the neuropsychologist who needs to identify changes in cognitive function in particular individuals.

Advances in pathophysiology in emergency and intensive care, and technological progress throughout medicine enable us to provide a highly professional clinical service for the severely ill. In the case of brain haemorrhage or an ischaemic infarct the diagnosis can be made immediately with the CT scan, and we have the techniques for reducing brain swelling, restoring both the cerebral circulation and cellular respiration. Fast intervention means a better chance of saving life and minimizes chronic disablement. The acute phase of the stroke lasts a few weeks during which strategies for rehabilitation of the patient have already been brought into play. For many reasons the methods used in rehabilitation of the elderly are different from those used with younger subjects. After a few months of treatment the patient must go back home, since the goal of rehabilitation is the resumption of the patient's former way of life. Here, the importance of social involvement emerges. Once discharged from hospital, a patient with a chronic disability risks the aggravation of his neurological signs if adequate follow-up assistance is not provided. Without it there is a vicious circle which leads to depression, lack of motivation and hypomobility. Spasticity may increase and new complications may arise, including ankylosis and bedsores. The patient ends up going back to hospital, not to the same rehabilitative centre, but to a long-stay institution. There is the risk that he will spend the rest of his life there, so defeating the work and the cost of the first hospital admission. We have taken the example of a stroke because this eventuality is frequent in the aged, as indicated by the distribution curve of admissions as a function of age in specialized centres for rehabilitation. Of a random sample of 4000 admissions to American hospitals, 15% of the aged were re-admissions and they represented a drain of two-thirds of the total annual cost (Gruenberg and Tompkins, 1985). This is an enormous proportion of the expenditure for such a small percentage of patients. Again in the USA, $8 billion is spent annually on aged patients who are re-admitted after 60 days (Collard, 1985).

It is not possible within this book to survey the hospital movements of the aged, because clinical and social practices differ so much from country to country and even from region to region. Even the legitimacy of the geriatric ward is still controversial. Some feel that their existence is not justified, both because the pathology is basically a branch of general medicine and because when wards are made up only of aged, mostly bedridden, patients it leads to discrimination. The word 'laager' is often applied. Others, especially geriatricians, hold that the aged need different organizational methods and equipment and that elderly patients might feel alienated and left out among younger people. The lack of general agreement is quite evident in countries like Italy, where the regions are free to decide for themselves. In some areas geriatric wards have been abolished, in others they still exist, while in some places they were never established.

The situation in Great Britain, where assistance for older people has a long tradition, is described by Hodkinson (1981). The model of care adopted in Great Britain is somewhat different from that of non-Anglo-Saxon countries. The majority of hospitalized patients in geriatric wards are discharged to their own home and only a few are transferred to old people's homes. The rate of discharge is reported to be the same for both sexes, though it is my experience, as I have pointed out in another part of the book, that it is more difficult to discharge older women. One of the fundamental causes is the patriarchal idea, that the head of the family should not be abandoned in the hospital.

Discharging a patient is an exercise of multi-disciplinary planning starting with case conferences on the ward. Doctors, nurses, therapists and social workers exchange information in order to come to the best arrangement for the patient. The proposed accommodation is visited and the patient has the opportunity to express his opinion. Contacts are made with relatives and friends in order to guarantee support and help. Many hospitals have a specific geriatric health visitor, who participates in the ward meetings and checks the progress of arrangements that have been made for the patient after discharge and requests further help as it is needed. In the absence of this supervision, one can imagine how easy it is for a relapse to occur and the benefits of treatment to be lost.

In the USA there is concern at the high proportion of admissions to hospital that do not produce lasting benefits despite the progressive approach to the care of the elderly. The problem is such that the pre-admission levels of disability are regained only months after discharge (Warshaw, 1985). The passage from cure to care is still in its infancy even in the USA (Loebel and Eisdorfer, 1984) with a lack of planned intervention and controlled evaluation. The importance of the multidisciplinary approach is stressed in America. This includes the involvement of administrative services, general and specialized doctors and medical services, nursing assistance, pharmacists, dietitian, dentist, occupational therapy, speech therapy, audiology, respiratory therapy, radiology, religious and recreational activities, hairdresser, beautician, social assistance, education, relatives and friends. How these agencies work together is 'easier to describe than to prescribe'. Even in the USA the problem of the leader in this group is considered crucial (Clark and Bray, 1984). A lack of effective leadership divides the various services into dissenting separate units, when order and structure are needed. Time and energy should not be wasted to the detriment of the patients. A great deal of debate is devoted to the different ways to lead a group, from authoritarian to tolerant, and on the characteristics desirable in the leader's personality. Clark and Bray emphasize the need to work harmoniously 'with reciprocal and fundamental acceptance of the right for each discipline to take part in the rehabilitative process'. This statement reveals the presence of tensions in many multi-disciplinary environments, including that of rehabilitation, because of group dynamics and different categories of interest. For example, in some places rehabilitation therapists claim their right to treat their patients autonomously, while elsewhere this takes place under medical supervision. For example, within the USA the therapist is independent in California, but is not so in Pennsylvania.

Even at the various intervention levels 'from cure to care' there exists discontinuity between significant stages of the patient's rehabilitation. Criticism has been made against this system, influenced by the institute needs and not by the patients, who are often dismissed not in order to begin a rehabilitative programme, but just to free a bed. On top of all this, there are enormous difficulties for long-term rehabilitation treatments which are covered for only a short time by federal subsidies and private insurance (Silverstone, 1984). In the USA too, there are serious problems for older persons hit by stroke. Few hospitals have staff specializing in hemiplegic recovery and there is often a long distance from the patient's home, so that they are often treated in clinics which are not really suitable (Hirschberg, 1976). Rehabilitation and social readjustment should re-install the individual's health and place in society, or at least minimize the damage. This is the citizen's right: we should add 'years to life and life to years' (Kottke, 1974).

The cost of looking after elderly patients in the USA has been calculated (at 1972 prices) as follows: patients not self-sufficient $8,300, patients at least capable of feeding themselves $4,600, figure dropping to $2,400 for those who are completely self-sufficient, but still need food and lodging (Kottke, 1974). In the USA expenditure on health care for the aged accounted for 33% of the total health bill, even when the percentage of the aged was about 11%. In 1981 the figure surpassed $83 billion with an average individual cost of $3,200 per year (Binstock, 1985). Health care costs have inflated at a greater rate than the general rate of inflation. Thus, the high cost of treatment is a cause for concern; politicians and administrators should ensure that it is repaid by high efficiency in management and their use of resources. There are serious difficulties regarding the financial contribution required from the aged themselves and their families. The figures of the Bureau of Census indicate that elderly people without relatives (who account for one third of the aged) have less than three fifths of the income of unrelated younger subjects. The average income of the aged is higher than that of families headed by people under 45 years of age, and less than that of families with older heads (Grad, 1984). The problem of poverty in old age strikes women hardest, not only because of their longer life span, but also because of the social treatment of widows, at least in the USA (Warlick, 1985).

Indeed, the problems of poverty are there even for the elderly who are not hypochondriac, and not beset with frequent trivial complaints, whose treatment is costly to the system. In the words of Goethe's Faust: 'however I dress I shall feel the pain of such a miserly existence'.

An intermediate form of assistance midway between hospitalization and community care is provided in the shape of the Day Hospital. In many cases these enable patients to receive necessary assistance without being withdrawn from the support of friends and family, but there is the possibility of a new confinement to the hospital (Hodkinson, 1981). If the degree of invalidity is not serious then day hospitals provide a valid alternative to hospitalization, but they should not be used as centres for follow-up after recovery instead of proper facilities for community health care. For this reason they have not been successful in many countries. The essential alternative to hospitalization is community health care. Under the guidance of a general physician, a team of nurses is assigned to the care of the patient in his own home. Technical procedures are carried out, including injections, phlebotomy, medication, enemas, bathing and general care. Besides this, other services are needed, including help with housework, bed-making, changing bed linen, preparation of a meal, possibly the provision of a hot meal at home, dressing, nutrition, the general toilet, help with correspondence and physical therapy. It is also important to ensure that the patient has company; a social life and help with personal affairs is needed. The incontinence of non-hospitalized patients is one of the most difficult disturbances for families to deal with: 97% of families view it as a great problem and 63% of the patients share the same feeling (Mohide and Pringle, 1985). A study conducted on 2,850 subjects who received community care revealed that 22% are incontinent. These have an average age of 81 and the majority of them (68%) are female, 50% are mentally deteriorated, 40% receive help with transport and 74% with mobility. Pads are used to deal with incontinence in 61% and only 9% are treated with drugs.

Self-sufficient patients who live on their own rather than with a younger family present important problems of compliance, that is to say, their success in following instructions for the use of medications (Macdonald and Macdonald, 1982). Drug prescriptions must therefore be clearly legible and intelligible with exact instructions on times and doses. The container/package must be easy to open. The patient must be instructed in his regimen and doctor to patient communications must be brief, with specific repeated recommendations. Knowledge of illness has not improved compliance. The doctor himself must imagine the possibility of unsatisfactory compliance. The number of drugs must be kept to the indispensable minimum and clinical checks must be frequent, even if it involves different doctors. The incidence of compliance varies among elderly subjects. If compliance is assessed by interview and the definition is 'taking drugs correctly', values of 70–85% are obtained. But, if it is measured by pill counting and the definition is 'taking between 50% and 200% of the prescribed tablets', compliance is observed in only 25% of outpatients (Macdonald and Macdonald, 1982).

Even though the cost of looking after a patient at home may be less than treating him in hospital, the facilities for community care are poorly developed in most places. In some countries, such as Italy, there are many general hospitals, but of a traditional nature, without proper provision for the aged. The stretched budgets of these institutions do not allow the hiring of new specialists and the retraining of existing staff poses problems, not least because it touches personal interest. In some places, union agreements greatly reduce the flexibility on matters like staff duties and movements. Thus it may happen that there is overstaffing in wards with few patients, while elsewhere it is not possible to employ sufficient nurses to care for hundreds of aged people with different degrees of invalidity.

To the lay person hospitalization means illness, but this is not always the case. In some countries it is common for hospital treatment to be motivated also by family, practical necessity and opportunism. For example, the apartments in some areas of summer resorts are rented to tourists, while the regular occupants find temporary housing elsewhere and the grandparents are sent to hospital under the pretext of a check-up. In large cities where younger members of the family work all day, the elderly parents remain at home alone for many hours each day. For them the hospital is a safe place where they can find assistance and company. From the clinician's point of view, it is very difficult to discharge an older person if the family is reluctant to have him at home. In my experience, family members fall into five categories of obstructionism: the humanitarian, the victim, the procrastinator, the jurist and the VIP. The humanitarian praises the hospital treatment received by his relative and does not want to deprive him of this great advantage. The victim lists a series of incredible financial and health problems which prevent him resuming responsibility for his relative. The procrastinator promises to make suitable arrangements for the relative, and after a long lapse of time announces a whole new scheme. The jurist pretends to know the current laws, holds that discharge cannot be imposed by the doctors and threatens charges. The VIP seeks the support of influential people whose authoritative intervention is intended to stop the doctor from discharging the elderly patient.

Such examples are common, especially in State-run hospitals. But, behind individual cases, there is a serious lack of an external planning and a crisis in our post-industrialized society. In the 1970s Franco Foschi, then Italy's Vice-Minister of Health, had already understood the weight of the problem. He said that: 'by now one generally recognizes that the conventional plans of organization are insufficient and wrong, inhumane, and unjust. In addition to this, the changes in our customs, in the role of the family and in the organization of society will lead to an increase in the selfish tendency which rejects the elderly. We must reject the move towards separate provision for the elderly, with coldly specialised social and health services: after all, they are full citizens of our society'.

As we have seen, sex differences in survival have important repercussions in the day-to-day life of elderly people, and even influence life conditions. Among the aged in the USA in 1978, 16% of the men and 40% of the women (the latter being more than 5.5 million) were living by themselves. The number of women living in the family is continuing to diminish. These figures reveal the importance of reducing premature male deaths and improving living conditions for older women (Brody, 1984).

In Great Britain, two thirds of the aged live in the family (Hodkinson, 1981). They often need a great deal of help from their relatives. The number of elderly people who have to be hospitalized because of significant physical or mental disabilities is much lower than among those who live alone, largely because of the sacrifices of their relatives. As a result large families do not always place the greatest demands on State-aided assistance, since the various children take it in turns to look after the elderly. In general it is the youngest unmarried daughter who takes care of the father (as did Antigone for Oedipus and Cordelia for King Lear). Now and then, living together creates problems, especially over different mental outlooks, and unconscious aggressiveness is directed toward elderly relatives who seek to limit personal freedom or who do not want to renounce their past role.

Many older people are proud of their independence and prefer to live alone. However, this choice has its own problems. The home, once well equipped and comfortable, becomes old and inadequate, cold and damp, in need of repair and modern sanitary fixtures. Narrow staircases and upper floors without lifts become obstacles for the aged. Moving house to more suitable accommodation is a problem too because it may mean moving to a new locality to find something modern and comfortable. In this case, elderly people may have to change their environment. In large cities this means going to an anonymous, suburban, dormitory area, away from old friends, where people do not know one another and where it is necessary to use public transport.

Sheltered housing, usually with resident helpers, is frequently advocated because of its advantages for older people who have difficulty coping in their old homes or in the lonely city outskirts, and who refuse the institutional care of an old people's home. Sheltered housing best takes the form of small apartments with a minimum of communal activity but help and assistance when needed, not too far from their home area. Shared housing systems have some disadvantages such as the often annoying duties imposed by the residents and management. In spite of this, 58–70% of 97 people interviewed, whose ages ranged from 54 to 97, claimed to be satisfied with the social advantages, safety, assistance, economy, freedom and lifestyle provided by this form of accommodation (West, 1985).

Today, health care is often provided by large medical complexes which include a primary care centre, an acute care hospital, a nursing home, a psychiatric hospital and a chronic care hospital, together furnishing a complete cradle-to-tomb service (Bulger, 1985). Such large systems make for savings in management costs due to the economies of scale and avoidance of duplication.

New initiatives are on the horizon, which will depend a great deal on philanthropy. In Italy, for example, the cost of health care will amount to $35 billion in 1986. It is not enough to meet public demand and aspirations and new initiatives will therefore depend largely on the intervention of benefactors. A political observer (Bertolini, personal communication) points out that there is a thriving development of volunteer aid. Indeed thanks to this, many young people are thought to have avoided drug addiction. The younger generation's maturity and drive shows that the desire for giving can replace the desire for receiving. In well-managed senior citizen centres, young and elderly volunteers play an active role in providing mental stimulation, education, physical and sporting activities, project work and political management, all of which help to create an environment of support and social relations once provided by the family. The work itself is important not so much for any monetary reward, as for moral gratification. Such rewards to a retired person for his service are more effective than anti-depressant therapy. I remember a distinguished gentleman, once the manager of a chemical firm, who acquired a new lease of life at St George's school in Venice explaining the history and art of Carpaccio, and helping visitors. The return for him was to feel alive and useful.

Retirement reduces enthusiasm, as well as the satisfaction of living. It may cause delusion and disappointment, especially in the second year (Ekerdt et al., 1985). In the USA out of 22.5 million older people not in hospital, 16% still work and 11% are actively mobile (Kirasic and Allen, 1985). Even a vacation project is important for the aged, especially if it can be enjoyed out of the main holiday season. Places with dry climates and winter temperatures higher than average, little wind, a railway station and possibly an airport, and communities rich in tradition, are ideal vacation sites for the elderly. They need to avoid places where the cold may cause illnesses. It is possible to create villages for the self-sufficient aged in these areas, fully equipped with services, designed by architects, psychologists, doctors and urban planners and tailored to the needs of their inhabitants:

pedestrian islands without steps or curbs, modular home nuclei, community restaurants, an outpatient centre, a religious centre, a cinema, theatre, gym, sports field, library, printing-works and other workshops. Regular transport to the historical town centre is important psychologically to avoid the feeling of isolation. The community needs to manage its own affairs and lead its own life. It must decide upon the form of village life, its amusements, cultural and sporting activities. The period spent in the community, meeting and knowing one another and creating activities can stimulate, interest and promote psychomotricity in a way that cannot be achieved in the fast and often violent lifestyle of a modern city. The cost of providing all this can be kept reasonably low, because the aged can pay for themselves or receive subsidies from State funds. A healthy aged person costs much less than a hospitalized one. Private and public enterprises may include in the contracts of their workers special contributions for the lodging of their older relatives. Consider, for example, a very modern community being developed by Father Ferlauto in Sicily, in perfect climatic conditions (Fig. 13.1). The religious approach and faith engender a serene attitude towards the future, removing the spectre of death and giving the elderly a strength to bear their present problems. In many older people one sees the sudden emergence of a mysticism that was perhaps suppressed in earlier years. In my view Dante's allegory in which old age (represented by St Bernard) allows one to rise up to God is appropriate to describe the positive aspects of being old (see Chapter 1). During the course of life, religious feelings become stronger especially in those already religious and there is a relationship, even if not a very strong one, between religiousness and satisfaction in life (Hunsberger, 1985; Markides, 1983). The fear of death depends neither on age nor on the nearness of the last day and men appear to suffer more than women (Maiden and Walker, 1985; Kiser, 1985). There may also be age differences in the sorrow experienced by elderly subjects when a relative dies (Davies and Hulligan, 1985).

Recommendation No. 779 of the European Council in 1976 concerning the rights of the patient states that the medical profession is at man's service and the prolonging of life must not be in and of itself the exclusive goal of medical practice. The doctor does not have the right even in cases which appear hopeless to rush the natural process of death, but nor should he act against the right of the ill person to avoid useless suffering. Euthanasia (*eu* = good and *thanatos* = death) is considered a crime of homicide under the majority of Penal Codes. It is considered as an aggravating circumstance when committed by a health care worker, while the patient's consent becomes an extenuating circumstance but does not exclude the crime. Medical ethics are very clear about this matter: no human life can be intentionally extinguished, even with good intention. Yet, in the case of an unfavourable prognosis, the doctor may limit his actual work to nutrition, pain therapy and moral assistance without heroic deeds.

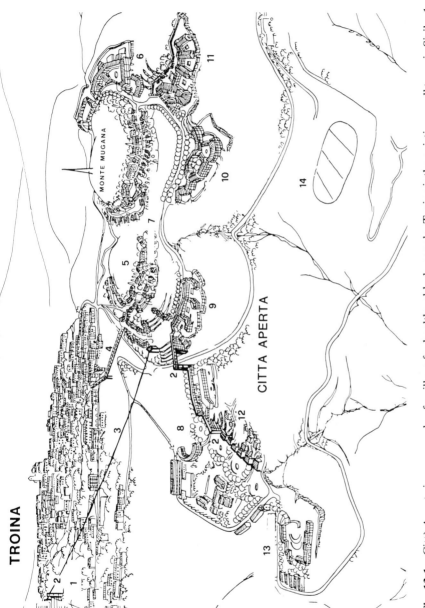

Fig. 13.1 Città Aperta is an example of a village for healthy elderly people. Troina is the existing small town in Sicily. 1 = administration centre and public services, 2 = elevators, 3 = cable tramway, 4 = bridge, 5 = residential area for families, 6 = study centre, 7 = living accommodation, 8 = medical facilities, 9 = centre of gerontology, 10 = training and working centre, 11 = informatics, telematics and graphic arts, 12 = handcraft, 13 = social and cultural centres, 14 = sport and recreational area

REFERENCES

Binstock, R. H. (1985). Health care of the aging: trends, dilemmas, and prospects for the year 2000. In C. M. Gaitz and T. Samorajski (Eds), *Aging 2000: Our Health Care Destiny*. New York: Springer-Verlag, pp. 3–15.

Brody, J. A. (1984). Facts, projections, and gaps concerning data on aging. *Public Health Rep., 99*, 468–475.

Bulger, R. J. (1985). Old wine in new bottles: medical care for the elderly in the year 2000. In C. M. Gaitz and T. Samorajski (Eds), *Aging 2000: Our Health Care Destiny*. New York: Springer-Verlag, pp. 511–519.

Clark, G. S., and Bray, G. P. (1984). Development of a rehabilitation plan. In T. F. Williams (Ed.), *Rehabilitation in the Aging*. New York: Raven Press, pp. 125–143.

Collard, A. (1985). Readmissions of elderly patients to the acute hospital. *Gerontologist, 25* (Suppl.), 27.

Davies, A. D. M., and Hulligan, A. (1985). Perception of life stress events by older and younger women. *Percept. Motor Skill, 60*, 925–926.

Diana, R. (1983). Psychosomatic aspects of aging. In A. Agnoli, G. Crepaldi, P. F. Spano and M. Trabucchi (Eds), *Aging*, vol. 23, New York: Raven Press, pp. 147–156.

Ekerdt, D. J., Bossé, R., and Levkoff, S. (1985). An empirical test for phases of retirement: findings from the normative aging study. *J. Gerontol., 40*, 95–101.

Grad, S. (1984). Incomes of the aged and nonaged. *Soc. Secur. Bull., 47*, 3–17.

Gruenberg, L., and Tompkins, C. (1985). Repeated hospitalizations and chronic conditions: their contribution to health care costs among the elderly. *Gerontologist, 25* (Suppl.), 27.

Hirschberg, G. C. (1976). Ambulation and self-care are goals of rehabilitation after stroke. *Geriatrics, 31*, 61–65.

Hodkinson, H. M. (1981). *An Outline of Geriatrics*. London: Academic Press.

Hunsberger, B. (1985). Religion, age, life satisfaction, and perceived sources of religiousness: a study of older persons. *J. Gerontol., 40*, 615–620.

Kirasic, K. C., and Allen, G. L. (1985). Aging, spatial performance and spatial competence. In N. Charness (Ed.), *Aging and Human Performance*. New York: John Wiley & Sons, pp. 191–223.

Kiser, M. L. (1985). Investigation of the correlates age and religiosity and their relationship to fear of death in the elderly: a preliminary study. *Gerontologist, 25* (Suppl.), 125.

Kottke, F. J. (1974). Historia obscura hemiplegiae. *Arch. Phys. Med. Rehabil., 55*, 4–13.

Loebel, J. P., and Eisdorfer, C. (1984). Psychological and psychiatric factors in the rehabilitation of the elderly. In T. F. Williams (Ed.), *Rehabilitation in the Aging*. New York: Raven Press, pp. 41–57.

Macdonald, E. T., and Macdonald, J. B. (1982). *Drug Treatment in the Elderly*. New York: John Wiley & Sons.

Maiden, R., and Walker, G. (1985). Attitude toward death across the life span. *Gerontologist, 25* (Suppl.), 125.

Markides, K. S. (1983). Aging, religiosity, and adjustment: a longitudinal study. *J. Gerontol., 38*, 621–625.

Mohide, E. A., and Pringle, D. M. (1985). A survey of urinary incontinence among elderly patients receiving organized home health care. *Gerontologist, 25* (Suppl.), 138.

Silverstone, B. (1984). Social aspects of rehabilitation. In T. F. Williams (Ed.), *Rehabilitation in the Aging*. New York: Raven Press, pp. 59–79.

Warlick, J. L. (1985). Why is poverty after 65 a woman's problem? *J. Gerontol., 40*, 751–757.

Warshaw, G. (1985). Functional decline in the hospitalized elderly. *Gerontologist, 25* (Suppl.), 3.

West, S. L. (1985). Shared housing: residents' view of gain and losses. *Gerontologist, 25* (Suppl.), 11.

Williams, T. F. (1984). Introduction. Rehabilitation in the aging: philosophy and approach. In T. F. Williams (Ed.), *Rehabilitation in the Aging*. New York: Raven Press, pp. xiii–xvi.

CHAPTER 14

Conclusions

Nowadays, Science, Politics and the mass media are focusing their attention on aging, as never before. The elderly are the people of the nineties.

Thousands of years have not been sufficient for mankind to understand whether aging necessarily brings with it a mental decline. Recent progress in knowledge, instrumentation and testing has certainly clarified many ideas on a topic that is still open to discussion and advancement. The parallel studies of genetics, histology, neurochemistry, electrophysiology, neuropsychology and clinical neurology help us to understand many of the changes that take place in aging but they have not resolved the question of decline. Multidisciplinary approaches are thought to be the proper way to solve problems as complex as those of aging, and new findings support the effectiveness of this type of research towards new frontiers. We have seen in this book that narrow fields of study, such as the age-dependent changes of a single enzyme, and crude measurement of mental ability contribute little to our understanding of the aging process. The resolution of the scientific method should be neither too fine nor too unrefined.

A number of new trends have emerged during the present decade. Let us re-examine the biological literature. In the beginning, scientists were concerned chiefly with the negative aspects of aging: the decrease of brain weight and volume, variations in neurons and glia, the loss of dendrites, widening of sulci and ventricles, senile plaques, tangles, alterations in capillaries, the deposit of lipofuscin, aluminium, copper, iron and melanin. DNA acquires inaccessible loci. The immune system declines. Membranes become thicker and neurotransmitters decline. The most refined scientific techniques have been employed to catalogue the deleterious changes which take place during aging, however small. Many of the observations have suggested a link between aging and dementia (Table 14.1).

Table 14.1   Does Alzheimer's disease represent an exaggeration of normal aging?

Yes. Some conclusions from literature:

There are quantitative differences between AD/SD and aging on the basis of quantitative histological studies (Tomlinson et al., 1970; Henderson et al., 1980; DeKosky and Bass, 1982).

There is a strong cell loss in normal elderly: −50% at age 90 (Gilloteaux and Linz, 1984).

AD/SD patients and the normal aged both have a 17% brain weight loss compared to the normal young. The cell loss in frontal cortex of aged demented patients is not significantly different from that found in normal aged subjects (DeKosky and Bass, 1982).

Microscopic specimens from the elderly and patients with senile dementia show senile plaques and tangles (Tomlinson et al., 1970; DeKosky and Bass, 1982). Tangles are also present in hippocampal pyramids of normal aged brains (Terry, 1980). Thirty-eight out of 51 random autopsies showed plaques and tangles in middle-aged, non-AD/SD subjects (Ulrich, 1985).

The number of glial cells and small neurons is similar in AD/SD and normal aging (Terry and Davies, 1983).

Dendritic loss (especially in horizontal and basal components) is seen in normal aging and AD/SD, with only quantitative differences (Scheibel and Scheibel, 1975).

Normal aging, accelerated by various factors including disease, produces most clinical dementias (Drachman, 1983).

The loss of frontal choline acetyltransferase (CAT) activity in the normal elderly and the less severe decrement in late Alzheimer's dementia mean that there is no difference in frontal cortex CAT activity between the two groups after age 75 (DeKosky et al., 1985).

Catecholamine catabolism is induced by MAO, enzymes that increase in aging and more so in Alzheimer's dementia (Adolfsson et al., 1979; Carlsson et al., 1980; Oreland, 1984).

AD/SD is an exacerbation of susceptibility to visual masking typically associated with normal aging (Coyne et al., 1984).

Multimodal tests of memory show similar profiles in elderly and demented subjects (Omer et al., 1985).

In both AD/SD patients and normal elderly auditory verbal selective reminding is better preserved than visual spatial selective reminding (Muramoto, 1984).

If we move on to consider the contribution of electrophysiology and neuropsychology, very small differences are seen between the normal elderly and young subjects; in some cases the difference may not exist. First of all it appears that variance among elderly people is high, especially when education plays a role in performance. When subjects are equated for educational levels or when performance is measured in a familiar setting, age differences in cognitive performance are reduced or vanish. Cross-sectional studies may enhance the apparent differences between cohorts, while longitudinal studies reduce them. An attempt to resolve the methodological problems of longitudinal vs. cross-sectional studies is offered in the approach indicated by Schaie (1983), which combines both methods in a single framework, called 'cohort-sequential'. In this experimental design each cohort is followed for 10 years or longer. The ages of the initial cohorts overlap in order to differentiate cohort effects from aging effects. In the Aging Twins Study cognitive functions are maintained in non-paced tests at least until age 75 (Fig. 14.1) and probably there are hereditary factors in some of the Wechsler Scale

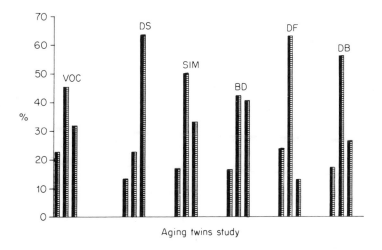

Aging twins study

Fig. 14.1 Longitudinal Aging Twins Study. The study began in 1946. On retest in 1955 each of the 78 subjects is labelled as increased (left), unchanged (centre) or decreased (right) for each of seven WAIS items: vocabulary (VOC), digit symbol (DS), similarities (SIM), block design (BD), digits forward (DF), digits backward (DB) and tapping (not shown here). Mean age of the subjects: 75.5 years. Nonpaced task performance is very stable. DS shows the greatest decrement. Adapted from Jarvik and Bank, 1983, with permission

factors. In fact, men decline more rapidly than women on tests of vocabulary, similarity and digit symbol substitution, which were found useful for the prediction of terminal decline and impending death (Jarvik and Bank, 1983). New data on the relative contribution of hereditary vs. external influences will be provided by the project on twins who were separated very early in their life and reared under different conditions (McClearn et al., 1985).

The performance of elderly subjects is not inferior to that of young controls in several areas of cognitive function including the perception of meaningful context, familiar problems, cued recall and previous experience. It is estimated that 90% of cognitive function is intact in old age (Kausler, 1982) and some mental processes, such as automatic attention and incidental learning are probably genetically protected. From all this, one can see that there is a need to fill the gap between laboratory tests and everyday life. A single parameter of measurement is not sufficient to characterize aging, whose understanding requires a knowledge of cognitive, affective and social behaviour with much more attention to the individual than to the group, as in the study of operant analysis.

The necessity for more ecological approaches to the study of aging does not cast doubt on the value of laboratory testing. On the contrary, such procedures are more likely to provide standardized normative data on aging and to clarify the processing of sensory information.

Electrophysiological investigation reveals that both stimulus-related and event-related potentials show only slight age-dependent changes in the latency of their components. The frequency of the EEG band undergoes a deceleration which, in the case of the alpha rhythm, is less than 1 Hz over a 50-year period. These findings provide evidence that psychological theories of a speed deficit in the elderly have a sound physical basis. The morphological differences between the young and the old are therefore accompanied by differences in performance and neurophysiology which are small or absent. The question is: is the picture different in dementia? Is dementia an exaggerated form of aging? The observations listed in Table 14.2 argue against this and indeed there is a growing feeling that aging and dementia are separate biological phenomena (Berg, 1985). There does appear to be a continuum between youth and aging, not between aging and dementia.

The fact that the phenomena of neurological aging are already present at age 30, as revealed by the CT scan studies, would probably come as an unpleasant surprise to people of that age who are active in their profession, sport and pastimes. To the layman, life is a parabolic arch from birth to the 70s, as the Bible says (Psalms 90,10):

Dies annorum nostrorum septuaginta anni
aut in valentibus octoginta anni
et maior pars eorum labor et dolor

(the days of our years are threescore and ten, or even by reason of strength fourscore years; yet is their pride but labour and sorrow).

Yet optimism stems from the recent observations of the stability of many brain functions and of the maintenance of neural plasticity. Homeostasis is maintained to a certain extent through the regeneration of dendrites and synapses and is favoured by environmental stimulation. Some enzymes and axonal terminals show regular cycles of regeneration. In many respects the mechanism of aging is similar to that of differentiation and growth. The gene regulation theory explains two important features of aging, i.e. 1) functional deterioration of specific brain areas and enzymes, 2) determination of life span. The gene regulation theory is

Table 14.2   Does Alzheimer's disease represent an exaggeration of normal aging?

No. Some conclusions from the literature.

If the effects of aging are similar to those of diffuse brain damage (including diseases of different aetiology), the magnitude of the difference should decrease with age. It does not (Goldstein and Shelly, 1975).

AD/SD patients dying before the age of 80 years tend to have diffuse brain atrophy. Over the age of 80 few demented patients show generalized atrophy beyond that due to aging and have temporal lobe atrophy (Hubbard and Anderson, 1981). Regression analysis does not show a significant decrease with age for the temporal region (Gibson, 1983).

In contrast to normal aging AD/SD is associated with a decrease in large cortical neurons and a four-fold increase in fibrous astrocytes in layers 2–6 (Terry and Davies, 1983).

Not all histological age-related changes are advanced in AD/SD and Down's syndrome (Mann et al., 1984a).

Selective dendritic growth exists in normal aging even at age 90, but this process is lost in AD/SD (Buell and Coleman, 1981).

In 90 year olds, the cortical changes in those with AD/SD are similar to those who have undergone normal aging alone (Mann et al., 1984b). This plateau should not exist, if dementia were exaggerated aging (Berg, 1985).

Brain metabolism ($CMRO_2$ and CMR_{glc}) is unaffected by normal aging (see Table 6.1, this book) in contrast to AD/SD.

Choline acetyltransferase (CAT) decreases in AD/SD independently of the age-dependent, physiological trend (Sorbi et al., 1980; Carlsson, 1985).

Mean alpha frequency is only slightly decreased in the normal elderly (see Table 7.6, this book) and the scalp distribution of this rhythm is preserved (Giaquinto and Nolfe, 1986). The EEG power spectrum undergoes different changes in demented patients.

Language is unaffected in normal aging and can even improve, in contrast to its fate in AD/SD (e.g., Goldstein, 1980; Gainotti et al., 1980; O'Dowd, 1983; Bandera et al., 1985; Poitrenaud et al., 1983). AD/SD is associated with a pattern of linguistic deficits that cannot be accounted for by existing models of aphasia (Emery, 1985).

The Halstead Battery indicates a clear difference between normal aging and brain damage, because some tests (Rhythm, Speech, Time Visual and Tapping) are sensitive to brain damage, but insensitive to normal aging. These tests explore the ability to perceive rhythmic patterns, to perceive consonants, to estimate time intervals and to perform fast and repetitive movements (Schludermann et al., 1983).

Spatial memory performance declines progessively with aging in normal subjects. Dementia is accompanied by an additional and separate decrement in spatial memory (Giaquinto et al., 1985).

The Rey verbal test reveals a similar learning curve in normal young and elderly subjects. The learning curve is flattened in demented patients (Giaquinto et al., 1985).

In the normal elderly, memory performance is only mildly impaired on tasks of effortful recollection. This memory is helped if the tasks and cues are familiar. AD/SD patients are seriously impaired on tasks of effortful recollection and are not helped by the familiarity of the cues. In some respects their memory resembles that of infants (Moscovitch, 1985).

---

supported by the fact that aging processes seem to affect men more than women (Table 14.3).

Cognitive rehabilitation is important for reducing age-differences and even for improving performance beyond the normal range. After 30 training sessions in

Table 14.3   Sex-differences among elderly people. Some statements from the literature.

Features favouring females

In aging twins study women outscore men on vocabulary, similarities and digit-symbol substitution. These tests are also useful in predicting critical loss and impending death (Jarvik and Bank, 1983).

Higher life expectancy (WHO, 1984).

Lower Brain Index Atrophy at CT scan (Takeda and Matsuzawa, 1984).

Preferential perfusion of the frontal and prefrontal regions (hyperfrontality) has a better stability in women (Mamo et al., 1983).

In longitudinal Aging Twin Studies women outscore men on most of the psychological tests administered (Jarvik and Bank, 1983).

Better comprehension without the speaker's face visible and in noise (Obler et al., 1985).

Higher average gains for the lowest test frequencies in vestibulo-ocular testing (Wall et al., 1984).

Better olfactory discrimination (Doty et al., 1984).

Lower hearing loss (Verrillo and Verrillo, 1985).

Less delta and more beta activity in the EEG (Wang and Busse, 1969; Giaquinto and Nolfe, 1986). Gender disparity also at younger ages (Shearer et al., 1984).

Shorter latencies of I and VII peaks in brain stem responses, some shorter interpeak lags and higher amplitude of the peaks (Nai-Shin Chu, 1985). Pontine conduction of auditory system is faster (Allison et al., 1984).

Variations in visual evoked potentials associated with increasing age are less evident in women (Allison et al., 1984). Gender differences are also reported in the sensory evoked potential, since N20 and P25 latencies in women are about 0.40 msec shorter (Simpson and Erwin, 1983).

The latency of the visual evoked potential is shorter (Allison et al., 1984).

The latency of P3 response is 17 msec shorter (Mullis et al., 1985).

Women maintain sleep better than men, have longer stage 3 and greater phasic REM activity (Reynolds et al., 1985).

In 100 couples the wife's memory for proper names was better in 80%, the husband's in 12% and were about equal in 8% (Miller Fisher, 1985).

Features favouring males

In a vocabulary test, males score significantly higher and give more good explanations (O'Dowd, 1983).

Males have a better performance in perspective-taking skills and in matching rotated blocks (Berg et al., 1982; Herman and Bruce, 1983).

Men have superior mechanical skill and shorter reaction times (Welford, 1985).

---

experiments of self-paced learning, elderly subjects can normally recall 30 words in their original order at the first trial. A 70-year-old man has recalled 120 figures in a row, an astonishing performance (Baltes and Kliegl, 1986). Mental exercise probably protects against cognitive decline and a positive relationship between continuous mental activity and successful aging probably exists (Jarvik and Bank, 1983).

Creativity can remain high even in very old age. Table 14.4 displays examples

Table 14.4   Famous long-lived Renaissance painters

	Dates	Age at death (years)
Tiziano	1477–1576	99
Giambellino	1425–1516	91
Michelangelo	1475–1564	89
Paolo Uccello	1397–1475	78
Luca Signorelli	1445–1523	78
Andrea Mantegna	1431–1506	75
Il Perugino	1448–1523	75
Piero della Francesca	1420–1492	72

of creativity and longevity in Renaissance painters. There is no trace of decline in their art until death. The elderly artist may be impaired by motor disturbances, not by cognitive ones. Dante says '. . . like the artist who has the shape in his mind and a trembling hand' (*Paradiso,* XIII, 78).

Following so many promising results with neuropsychological training and the examples of creativity at old age, let us consider the controversial issue of so-called cognitive drugs. Many scientists and clinicians deny a present or future role for pharmacological intervention in cases of mental decline. Knowledge in this field has grown continuously for the last 20 years. This period is nothing, if we consider four centuries elapsed between the birth of chemistry, with Paracelsus, and the discovery of the first anti-epileptic molecule. The great neurologists of last century, like Charcot and Dejerine and Hughlings Jackson certainly experienced no success in treating epileptic patients, many of whom are nowadays successfully cured.

The health of elderly people receives more serious consideration today than it has done in the past. Perhaps the recent interest in this issue is not pure philanthropy but a sign of the anguish of a society which is becoming old. Hopefully, closer collaboration between biologists, clinicians, sociologists and politicians will improve the quality of life for the old. New forms of care which provide respect for human dignity, a serene but active lifestyle, meaningful roles and responsibilities, and the prevention of disease will be the general issues of the near future. It is likely that improvement in primary care will be developed on the basis of better host defences, involving the technology of monoclonal antibodies for diagnosis and treating tumours (Bulger, 1985). From this point of view chronic diseases are seen more as expressions of host failure than as the penetration of external agents (Birren, 1985). Stopping smoking is highly recommended by the

WHO, no matter at what age. Severe hypertension must be treated in all cases, whereas mild forms require no mandatory pharmacological intervention since that may bring about side-effects. Lifestyle must be improved for this segment of society. The architecture of buildings and roads, as well as transportation require special care to avoid risks for the elderly. Travelling should be encouraged: some countries, like Italy, issue a special card which secures large discounts on railways and in theatres.

The epidemiological approach supplies the data for programming and evaluating the demographic, social and economic characteristics of a population. It also makes it possible to monitor health conditions in the country, public facilities, results and their costs. For many years the inadequate allocation of health resources has been denounced in many countries. A WHO statement indicates that 'the services provided are often geared more to the bureaucratic structure of the provider than to the needs of the user' (WHO, 1984). Scientific observations should not be confined to meetings and journals but must be considered by the politicians and the managers of social welfare planning. If the final goal of a proper service is missed, most of our scientific observations will prove to have been elegant but vain academic activities.

REFERENCES

Adolfsson, R., Gottfries, C. G., Ross, B. E., and Winblad, B. (1979). Postmortem distribution of dopamine and homovanillic acid in human brain, variations related to age and a review of the literature. *J. Neural Transm.*, 45, 81–105.

Allison, T., Hume, A. L., Wood, C. C., and Goff, W. R. (1984). Development and aging changes in somatosensory, auditory and visual evoked potentials. *Electroenceph. Clin. Neurophysiol.*, 58, 14–24.

Baltes, P. B., and Kliegl, R. (1986). On the dynamics between growth and decline in the aging of intelligence and memory. In K. Poeck, H. J. Freund and H. Gaenshirt (Eds), *Neurology*. Berlin: Springer-Verlag, pp. 1–17.

Bandera, R., Capitani, E., Della Sala, S., and Spinnler, H. (1985). Discrimination between senile dementia Alzheimer type patients and education matched normal controls by means of a 6-test set. *Ital. J. Neurol. Sci.*, 6, 339–344.

Berg, L. (1985). Does Alzheimer's disease represent an exaggeration of normal aging? *Arch. Neurol.*, 42, 737–739.

Berg, C., Hertzog, C. K., and Hunt, E. (1982). Age differences in the speed of mental rotation. *Dev. Psychol.*, 18, 95–107.

Birren, J. E. (1985). Health care in the 21st century: the social and ethical context. In C. M. Gaitz and T. Samorajski (Eds) *Aging 2000: Our Health Care Destiny*. New York: Springer-Verlag, pp. 521–530.

Buell, S. J., and Coleman, P. D. (1981). Quantitative evidence for selective dendritic growth in normal human aging but not in senile dementia. *Brain Res.*, 214, 23–41.

Bulger, R. J. (1985). Old wine in new bottles: medical care for the elderly in the year 2000. In C. M. Gaitz and T. Samorajski (Eds) *Aging 2000: Our Health Care Destiny*. New York: Springer-Verlag, pp. 511–519.

Carlsson, A. (1985). Brain neurotransmitter in normal aging. In C. M. Gaitz and T. Samorajski (Eds) *Aging 2000: Our Health Care Destiny*. New York: Springer-Verlag, pp. 113–122.

Carlsson, A., Gottfries, C. G., Svenner-Holm. L., Adolfsson, R., Oreland, L., Winblad,

B., and Aquilonius, S. M. (1980). Neurotransmitters in human brain analyzed post mortem: changes in normal aging senile dementia and chronic alcoholism. In U. K. Rinne, M. Klinger, G. Stamm (Eds), *Parkinson's Disease*. New York: Elsevier-North Holland, pp. 121–133.

Coyne, A. C., Liss, L., and Geckler, C. (1984). The relationship betwen cognitive status and visual information processing. *J. Gerontol.*, 39, 711–717.

DeKosky, S. T., and Bass, N. H. (1982). Aging, senile dementia and the intralaminar microchemistry of cerebral cortex. *Neurology*, 32, 1227–1233.

DeKosky, S. T., Scheff, S. W., and Markesbery, W. R. (1985). Laminar organization of cholinergic circuits in human frontal cortex in Alzheimer's disease and aging. *Neurology*, 35, 1425–1431.

Doty, R. L., Shaman, P., Applebaum, S. L., Giberson, R., Siksorski, L., and Rosenberg, L. (1984). Smell identification ability: changes with age. *Science*, 226, 1441–1443.

Drachman, D. A. (1983). How normal aging relates to dementia: a critique and classification. In D. Samuel, S. Algeri, S. Gershon, V. E. Grimm and G. Toffano (Eds), *Aging*, vol. 22. New York: Raven Press, pp. 19–31.

Emery, O. B. (1985). Language and aging. *Exp. Aging Res.*, 11, 3–60.

Gainotti, G., Caltagirone, C., Masullo, G., and Miceli, G. (1980). Patterns of neuropsychological impairment in various diagnostic groups of dementia. In L. Amaducci, A. N. Davison and P. Antuono (Eds), *Aging*, vol. 13. New York: Raven Press, pp. 245–250.

Giaquinto, S., and Nolfe, G. (1986). The EEG in the normal elderly: a contribution to the interpretation of aging and dementia. *Electroenceph. Clin. Neurophysiol.*, 63, 540–546.

Giaquinto, S., Nolfe, G., and Calvani, M. (1985). Cluster analysis of cognitive performance in elderly and demented subjects. *Ital. J. Neurol. Sci.*, 6, 157–165.

Gibson, P. H. (1983). EM study of the numbers of cortical synapses in the brains of ageing people and people with Alzheimer-type dementia. *Acta Neuropathol. (Berlin)*, 62, 127–133.

Gilloteaux, J. and Linz, M. H. (1984). Histology of aging: central nervous system. *Gerontol. Geriat. Educat.*, 4, 81–97.

Goldstein, G. (1980). Psychopathological dysfunction in the elderly: discussion. In J. O. Cole and J. E. Barrett (Eds), *Psychopathology in the Aged*. New York: Raven Press, pp. 137–144.

Goldstein, G., and Shelly, C. H. (1975). Similarities and differences between psychological deficit in aging and brain damage. *J. Gerontol.*, 30, 448–455.

Henderson, G., Tomlinson, B. E., and Gibson, P. H. (1980). Cell counts in human cerebral cortex in normal adults throughout life using an image analysing computer. *J. Neurol. Sci.*, 46, 113–136.

Herman, J. F., and Bruce, P. R. (1983). Adults' mental rotation of spatial information: effects of age, sex and cerebral laterality. *Exp. Aging Res.*, 9, 83–85.

Hubbard, B. M., and Anderson, J. M. (1981). A quantitative study of cerebral atrophy in old age and senile dementia. *J. Neurol. Sci.*, 50, 135–145.

Jarvik, L. F., and Bank, L. (1983). Aging twins: longitudinal psychometric data. In K. W. Schaie (Ed.), *Longitudinal Studies of Adult Psychological Development*. New York: The Guilford Press, pp. 40–63.

Kausler, D. H. (1982). *Experimental Psychology and Human Aging*. New York: John Wiley & Sons.

Mamo, H., Meric, P., Luft, A., and Seylaz, J. (1983). Hyperfrontal pattern of human cerebral circulation. *Arch. Neurol.*, 40, 626–632.

Mann, D. M. A., Yates, P. O., and Marcyniuk, B. (1984a). Relationship between pigment accumulation and age in Alzheimer's disease and Down syndrome. *Acta Neuropathol. (Berlin)*, 63, 72–77.

Mann, D. M. A., Yates, P. O., and Marcyniuk, B. (1984b). Alzheimer's presenile dementia, senile dementia of Alzheimer type and Down's syndrome in middle age form an age related continuum of pathological changes. *Neuropathol. Applied. Neurobiol.,* 10, 185–207.

McClearn, G. E., Plomin, R., Pedersen, N. L., Friberg, L. T., deFaire, U., and Nesselroade, J. R. (1985). Genetic and environmental influences in behavioral aging: the swedish adoption/twin study of aging (SATSA). *Gerontologist,* 25, 104.

Miller Fisher, C. (1985). Vascular disease, senility, and dementia. *Lancet,* 8421, 173–174.

Moscovitch, M. (1985). Memory from infancy to old age: implications for theories of normal and pathological memory. *Ann. N.Y. Acad. Sci.,* 444, 78–96.

Mullis, R. J., Holcomb, P. J., Diner, B. C., and Dykman, R. A. (1985). The effects of aging on the P3 component of the visual event-related potential. *Electroenceph. Clin. Neurophysiol.,* 62, 141–149.

Muramoto, O. (1984). Selective reminding in normal and demented aged people: auditory verbal versus visual spatial task. *Cortex,* 20, 461–478.

Nai-Shin Chu (1985). Age-related latency changes in the brain-stem auditory evoked potentials. *Electroenceph. Clin. Neurophysiol.,* 62, 431–436.

O'Dowd, S. C. (1983). Vocabulary test performance of old and young adults: another look at quality scoring. *J. Gen. Psychol.,* 109, 167–180.

Obler, L. K., Nicholas, M., Albert, M. L., and Woodward, S. (1985). On comprehension across the adult lifespan. *Cortex,* 21, 273–280.

Omer, H., Babayov, D., and Menczel, J. (1985). Comparison of verbal and nonverbal memory in elderly normal subjects and dementia patients. *Isr. J. Med. Sci.,* 21, 283–287.

Oreland, L. (1984). Monoamine oxidase and normal aging and in AD/SDAT. *Clin. Neuropharmacol.,* 7 (Suppl. 1), 32–33.

Poitrenaud, J., Barrère, H., Darcet, P., and Driss, F. (1983). Le viellissement des fonctions cognitives. *Presse Mèd.,* 48, 3119–3123.

Reynolds III, C. F., Kupfer, D. J., Taska, L. S., Hoch, C. C., Sewitch, D. E., and Spiker, D. G. (1985). Sleep of healthy seniors: a revisit. *Sleep,* 8, 20–29.

Schaie, K. W. (1983). What can we learn from the longitudinal study of adult psychological development? In K. W. Schaie (Ed.), *Longitudinal Studies of Adult Psychological Development.* New York: The Guilford Press, pp. 1–19.

Scheibel, M. E., and Scheibel, A. B. (1975). Structural changes in the aging brain. In H. Brody, D. Harman and J. M. Ordy (Eds), *Aging,* vol. 1. New York: Raven Press, pp. 11–37.

Schludermann, E. H., Schludermann, S. M., Merryman, P. W., and Brown, B. W. (1983). Halstead's studies in neuropsychology of aging. *Arch. Gerontol. Geriat.,* 2, 49–172.

Shearer, D. E., Cohn, N. B., Dustman, R. E., and LaMarche, J. A. (1984). Electrophysiological correlates of gender differences: a review. *Amer. J. EEG Technol.,* 24, 95–107.

Simpson, D. M., and Erwin, C. W. (1983). Evoked potential latency change with age suggests differential aging of primary somatosensory cortex. *Neurobiol. of Aging,* 4, 59–63.

Sorbi, S., Antuono, P., and Amaducci, L. (1980). Choline acetyltransferase and acetylcholinesterase abnormalities in senile dementia: importance of biochemical measurements in human post-mortem brain specimens. *Ital. J. Neurol. Sci.,* 2, 75–83.

Takeda, S., and Matsuzawa, T. (1984). Brain atrophy during aging: a quantitative study using Computed Tomography. *J. Am. Geriat. Soc.,* 32, 520–524.

Terry, R. D. (1980). Structural changes in senile dementia of the Alzheimer type. In L. Amaducci, A. N. Davison and P. Antuono (Eds), *Aging,* vol. 13. New York: Raven Press, pp. 23–32.

Terry, R. D., and Davies, P. (1983). Some morphological and biochemical aspects of Alzheimer's disease. In D. Samuel, S. Algeri, S. Gershon, V. E. Grimm and G. Toffano (Eds), *Aging,* vol. 22. New York: Raven Press, pp. 47–59.

Tomlinson, B. E., Blessed, G., and Roth, M. I. (1970). Observations in the brains of demented old people. *J. Neurol. Sci.,* 11, 205–242.

Ulrich, J. (1985). Alzheimer changes in nondemented patients younger than sixty-five: possible early stages of Alzheimer's disease and senile dementia of Alzheimer type. *Ann. Neurol.*, 17, 273–277.

Verrillo, R. T., and Verrillo, V. (1985). Sensory and perceptual performance. In N. Charness (Ed.), *Aging and Human Performance*. New York: John Wiley & Sons, pp. 1–46.

Wall III, C., Black, F. O., and Hunt, A. E. (1984). Effect of age, sex and stimulus parameters upon vestibulo-ocular responses to sinusoidal rotation. *Acta Otolaryngol. (Stock.)*, 98, 270–278.

Wang, H. S., and Busse, E. W. (1969). EEG of healthy old persons — A longitudinal study. I. Dominant background activity and occipital rhythm. *J. Gerontol.*, 24, 419–426.

Welford, A. T. (1985). Changes of performance with age: an overview. In N. Charness (Ed.), *Aging and Human Performance*. New York: John Wiley & Sons, pp. 333–369.

World Health Organization (1984). The uses of the epidemiology in the study of the elderly. *Technical Reports Series* 706. Geneva.

Subject index